Catherine Kingcombe.

For W.B. Saunders

*Commissioning Editor* Ellen Green
*Project Editor* Jane Shanks
*Project Controller* Frances Affleck
*Design Direction* Sarah Cape

# MCQs in Paediatrics

### Edited by

## Tom Marshall FRCP
Royal Hospital for Sick Children, Edinburgh

## Dominic Cochran MRCP
Royal Hospital for Sick Children, Glasgow

## Louise Bath MRCP
Royal Hospital for Sick Children, Edinburgh

W. B. SAUNDERS

Edinburgh · London · New York · Philadelphia · Sydney · Toronto

W.B. SAUNDERS

An imprint of Harcourt Publishers Limited

© Harcourt Brace & Company Limited 1999
© Harcourt Publishers Limited 2000

First published 1999
 Reprinted 2000

ISBN 0-7020-2249-7

*British Library Cataloguing in Publication Data*
A catalogue record for this book is available from the British Library.

*Library of Congress Cataloging in Publication Data*
A catalog record for this book is available from the Library of Congress

Medical knowledge is constantly changing. As new information becomes
available, changes in treatment, procedures, equipment and the use of drugs
become necessary. The authors and the publishers have, as far as it is
possible, taken care to ensure that the information given in this text is
accurate and up to date. However, readers are strongly advised to confirm
that the information, especially with regard to drug usage, complies with
current legislation and standards of practice.

Typeset by LaserScript, Mitcham, Surrey
Printed in China

# Contents

# Introduction

The questions in this book have been compiled with the intention of covering the core Paediatric knowledge required by undergraduates. We have attempted to avoid more than passing reference to 'paediatric exotica'. Postgraduate students attempting the MRCPCH Part 1 exam should also find these questions a useful revision exercise.

The book consists of a variety of MCQ types: some factual, some data interpretation and some based on clinical problems. The latter require a certain amount of judgement or experience to answer.

We have adopted a systematic approach to the layout of questions in the book but have also included four 'minitests' throughout the book. The questions in the four mini-quizzes are of similar range and difficulty and should allow you to monitor your progress as you work your way through the book. At the end of the book, there is a 'blockbuster' test of 300 questions which you should complete under exam conditions.

Common problems recur in many different paediatric specialties. There are a few basic physiological disturbances which underpin many disease processes. You will therefore find that there is some repetition of clinical themes and physiological principles in different sections of the book. We make no apology for this and hope that revision and restatement of important points will aid the learning process.

There is a move among many of the examining bodies away from negative marking in MCQ exams, and away from peer-referenced marking (i.e. only the top 30% pass). This system is being replaced by criterion-referenced marking where all those reaching a given standard will pass, although the accepted standard (pass mark) may be set as high as 80% for an exam based on core knowledge. We would suggest that the test questions in this book should be answered under exam conditions. You should adapt your question answering technique according to the marking system which you are likely to encounter. With *no* negative marking, all questions should be attempted. However, if you are going to encounter a negative marking system for wrong answers, do not guess when you have no idea about the right answer! You may be able to answer some questions after consideration of the basic scientific principles. On other questions, if you have an idea of the correct answer, it may be a good idea to go with your hunches! Use this book to work out your best question answering technique, and to find out how reliable your hunches really are.

*Tom Marshall*

# Minitest 1

1. **In a 2-year-old with persistence of the ductus arteriosus:**
   A. the murmur is continuous with a systolic accentuation.
   B. there is a wide pulse pressure.
   C. the murmur quietens on lying the child down.
   D. the ductus will be closed by administration of indomethacin.
   E. there will be cyanosis on exercise.

2. ***First-line* treatment of mild flexural eczema in an 18-month-old infant would include:**
   A. a low-antigenic diet, including milk protein and egg exclusion.
   B. betamethasone cream applied four times daily for 1 week.
   C. regular application of antibiotic cream.
   D. avoidance of soap for washing.
   E. regular application of emulsifying ointment to affected areas.

3. **A 3-year-old child is admitted to A&E with a short history of a sore throat, pain on swallowing, high fever and a low-pitched grunting noise while breathing. The child appears toxic, is sitting forward and unable to swallow secretions. There is no significant cough and only mild chest recession. The following would be appropriate management:**
   A. carefully inspect the pharynx for evidence of tonsillitis or foreign body.
   B. insert an intravenous cannula to obtain blood samples and start IV fluids.
   C. send to X-ray for inspiratory and expiratory CXR to exclude a foreign body.
   D. ask the anxious parents to leave the room as they may upset the child.
   E. give oxygen.

4. **Children with the following medical problems are at increased risk of developing hypothyroidism:**
   A. Down syndrome.
   B. severe asthma requiring treatment with continuous oral steroids.
   C. diabetes mellitus.
   D. hydrocephalus.
   E. Turner syndrome.

1. **AB**

   The typical murmur of a persistent ductus arteriosus (PDA) is continuous with a systolic accentuation. The pulmonary artery pressure is usually low and there is therefore a rapid fall in aortic systolic pressure as blood shunts into the pulmonary circuit. There is a wide pulse pressure and the pulses may easily be felt. The fontanelle may be obviously pulsatile. The murmur does not quieten on lying down – this would be much more suggestive of a venous hum (with inspiratory accentuation). The defect can be closed only by indomethacin within the first 2 months of life, usually in preterm babies. There is no cyanosis with a PDA.

2. **DE**

   First-line treatment for *mild* eczema does not include dietary manipulation. Routine management includes regular use of moisturisers such as aqueous cream, use of bath oil and avoidance of soaps and bubble-baths, which will degrease the skin. Antibiotics are given, usually by mouth, only when there is evidence of infection (usually with Staphylococcus). Powerful fluorinated steroids are not used in young children with mild skin disease.

3. **E**

   This is a classical history of acute epiglottitis. In epiglottitis airway obstruction may occur at any time, particularly if the child is upset. Answers ABC or D – if put into clinical practice – could be regarded as constituting negligent practice. Children with airway obstruction usually collapse because of hypoxia. After hearing this typical history and observing the signs of airway obstruction, the parents should be encouraged to hold an oxygen mask as close to the child's face as tolerated. Oxygen saturation is monitored, and everyone should keep very calm and senior anaesthetic help (and ENT if necessary) summoned urgently.

4. **ACE**

   There is an association between chromosomal abnormality and hypothyroidism. Diabetic children are at risk of other auto-immune disorders, particularly hypothyroidism and coeliac disease. There is no relationship between asthma or hydro-cephalus and hypothyroidism.

5. **A 3-year-old child is reported by his mother to have an excessive thirst. On examination, the child appears healthy and is normally grown. You should:**
   A. carry out immediate urinalysis.
   B. measure 24 hour fluid balance.
   C. admit immediately to hospital for a careful water-deprivation test.
   D. request renal ultrasound and isotope scans.
   E. check an early morning urine osmolarity.

6. **The following stools are typical of the associated condition:**
   A. watery stool with visible vegetable material and toddlers' diarrhoea.
   B. oily stools and cystic fibrosis.
   C. explosive, watery stools and lactose intolerance.
   D. bloody diarrhoea and rotavirus gastroenteritis.
   E. constipation and Hirschsprung's disease.

7. **A conjugated hyperbilirubinaemia:**
   A. is suggested by jaundice with pale stools and dark urine.
   B. is caused by haemolysis.
   C. is caused by infectious hepatitis.
   D. is caused by biliary atresia.
   E. is significant only if the conjugated fraction is greater than 50% of the total bilirubin.

8. **The following conditions are caused by single gene defects:**
   A. Turner syndrome.
   B. Duchenne muscular dystrophy.
   C. cystic fibrosis.
   D. cleft lip.
   E. asthma.

5. **AE**

   The differential diagnosis includes an inability to concentrate urine, an osmotic diuresis or excessive fluid. Negative urinalysis will exclude diabetes mellitus and major renal pathology. A morning urine osmolarity of >600 mosm/kg obtained at home, without any fluid restriction, excludes a defect in urine concentrating ability. Simple habit is much the commonest cause of high fluid intake in young children.

6. **ABCE**

   Toddlers' diarrhoea is characterised by painless, watery stools which often contain vegetable matter. Affected infants thrive normally. Steatorrhoea stools are smelly due to undigested protein and fat. In cystic fibrosis the stools may be oily with visible fatty droplets. In sugar malabsorption large bowel bacterial fermentation of unabsorbed sugar results in an osmotic diarrhoea with excessive flatus production and an acid fluid stool. In Hirschsprung's disease there will be constipation, though if an enterocolitis develops, bloody diarrhoea may occur.

7. **ACD**

   A conjugated hyperbilirubinaemia is suggested by a greenish jaundice accompanied by pale stools (lack of bile pigment) and dark urine (bilirubinuria). Levels of conjugated bilirubin are significant if the conjugated fraction exceeds 20% of the total. Raised levels of conjugated bilirubin are found where there is anatomical obstruction to bile flow (e.g. biliary atresia), choledochal cyst or cystic fibrosis, or any functional obstruction with liver inflammation as in infective or metabolic hepatitis. Haemolysis causes an unconjugated hyperbilirubinaemia by exceeding the bilirubin conjugating ability of the liver.

8. **BC**

   Turner syndrome 45XO is a chromosomal abnormality. Duchenne muscular dystrophy is an X-linked recessive single gene defect. A number of mutations within the dystrophin gene have been described. Cystic fibrosis is an autosomal recessive condition – over 900 mutations have been described within this single large gene. Cleft lip and asthma are not single gene disorders, but have polygenic inheritance. In the case of asthma, there is also a very strong environmental element.

9. **A 13-month-old boy is not yet weightbearing. A reassuring line should be taken with the parents if:**
   A. the child is actively bottom shuffling.
   B. if lack of weightbearing is part of a pattern of more generalised delay in reaching milestones.
   C. if there is a family history of delayed walking in early infancy.
   D. if the child has already developed a clear hand preference.
   E. if muscle tone is generally reduced, but there is no other abnormality on neurodevelopmental examination.

10. **A normal 2-year-old child:**
    A. has a haemoglobin level of 15–20 g/dl.
    B. has a predominance of neutrophils over lymphocytes in the peripheral blood.
    C. has 25% fetal haemoglobin.
    D. will have an absolute neutrophil count of greater than $1.0 \times 10^9$/L.
    E. will have an MCV of greater than 90 fl.

11. **Babies born in the UK to mothers who are HIV antibody positive:**
    A. are considered to be HIV infected if they are HIV antibody positive at birth.
    B. should be breast-fed.
    C. have a less than 15% risk of being infected themselves.
    D. are at increased risk of neonatal sepsis.
    E. have a life expectancy of 6–12 months if HIV culture is positive.

9. **ACE**

   Bottom shuffling infants are often slower than average (13 months) at walking independently. There is commonly a family history of delayed walking, which is of reassurance. Benign central hypotonia is often associated with a delay in reaching gross motor milestones, but development is otherwise normal. Global delay should always be a cause for concern. A clear hand preference at 13 months should raise the possibility that the other hand has a disability – e.g. a hemiplegia. Hand preference usually develops after 18 months of age.

10. **D**

    Haemoglobin levels fall from 15–20 g/dl at birth to 10–11 g/dl at 3 months. There is a lymphocyte predominance in the peripheral blood until 4 years of age when a neutrophil-predominant picture takes over. Full-term neonates have 65% fetal Hb – levels fall to less than 5% by 3 months of age. An absolute neutrophil count of less than $1.0 \times 10^9/L$ represents significant neutropenia with a risk of spontaneous infection. The normal MCV is < 90 fl.

11. **C**

    Tests demonstrating *infection*, such as a positive HIV culture, are required for HIV diagnosis. HIV may be transmitted in breast milk. In the UK, HIV-infected mothers are advised not to breast-feed. In Africa, where infant mortality is high, breast feeding is advised even when the mother has HIV infection. In the UK rates of vertical HIV transmission are less than 15%. Life expectancy for babies born to HIV-positive mothers in good health is more than 10 years and is likely to increase further with the newer drug regimes. There is no increased risk of neonatal sepsis.

12. **A 10-year-old boy with insulin-dependent diabetes, on a twice daily routine of long- and short-acting insulins, reports regular hypoglycaemia while playing football in the afternoon. To prevent this problem recurring, you should advise him to:**
    A. give less short-acting insulin before breakfast.
    B. test his urine for sugar before playing football.
    C. give up playing football.
    D. take glucose tablets when he begins to feel lightheaded.
    E. eat extra carbohydrate, such as a small chocolate bar, before football.

13. **Results of investigations performed on *cerebrospinal fluid* from a febrile, irritable, 4-year-old are as follows: white cell count, 150 × 10$^9$/L; differential count, 50% lymphocytes, 30% neutrophils, 20% macrophages; protein 1.0 g/L, CSF glucose 0.8 mmol/L, blood glucose 5.0 mmol/L; and microscopy – no organisms seen. These results are compatible with a diagnosis of:**
    A. tuberculous meningitis.
    B. viral meningitis.
    C. untreated bacterial meningitis.
    D. partially treated bacterial meningitis.
    E. brain abscess.

14. **The following are more typical of the early physical examination findings of a premature than a post-term baby:**
    A. hypotonia.
    B. obvious plantar skin creases.
    C. prominent clitoris, not covered by labia.
    D. palpable breast buds.
    E. abundant lanugo hair.

15. **The following renal investigations would be appropriate:**
    A. an ultrasound scan to assess function.
    B. a DMSA isotope scan to assess presence of renal scarring.
    C. a Mag 3 isotope scan to assess vesico-ureteric reflux.
    D. a micturating cystourethrogram to assess vesico-ureteric reflux.
    E. an IVP to demonstrate the presence of an ectopic ureter.

**12. DE**

Less short-acting insulin in the morning will result in morning hyperglycaemia. A smaller dose of long-acting insulin given in the morning will result in a higher blood glucose in the afternoon before football. Exercise should be encouraged. All diabetic children should carry dextrose tablets to treat any episodes of symptomatic hypoglycaemia. A common strategy is to encourage children to take one or two extra carbohydrate exchanges (one exchange = 10 g carbohydrate) before exercise.

**13. ADE**

In TB meningitis there is often a long history. The CSF protein is raised with mostly lymphocytes on microscopy. In viral meningitis the CSF protein and sugar levels are usually normal. In bacterial meningitis the CSF sugar levels will be less than 50% of the blood sugar, the CSF protein levels will be raised and there will be mostly neutrophils on microscopy. In partially treated meningitis or brain abscess no organisms are seen usually on microscopy; there is a mixture of lymphocytes, neutrophils and macrophages on microscopy and a longer history. Lumbar puncture should not be performed if there are signs of raised intracranial pressure.

**14. ACE**

In order to determine the gestational age of neonates a number of superficial physical characteristics and neurological features mostly relating to muscle tone are assessed. Preterm babies tend to be hypotonic, have smooth skin, soft cartilage, undescended testes or prominent clitoris, abundant lanugo hair and no palpable breast tissue.

**15. BCDE**

Ultrasound will demonstrate the renal anatomy but gives little information about function. DMSA isotope is fixed in the renal tubules – 'cold' spots represent areas of non-functioning tissue or scarring. Mag 3 or DTPA isotopes are filtered by the glomeruli and give information about the speed of drainage and relative contribution of either kidney to overall function. By rescanning over the kidneys after micturition, it is possible to assess reflux in cooperative children over the age of 4 years. An MCU is the classical method of assessing vesico-ureteric reflux. An IVP gives anatomical information and demonstrates the position of an ectopic ureter – the kidney ultrasound scan may demonstrate a duplex collecting system.

16. **Simple absence seizure ('petit mal') epilepsy:**
    A.  is characterised by 3 cycles per second spike and wave EEG disturbance.
    B.  is effectively treated with ethosuxamide.
    C.  is provoked by hyperventilating.
    D.  attacks are followed by a period of sleepiness.
    E.  does not cause any disturbance of schoolwork.

17. **Migraine:**
    A.  symptoms begin before 10 years of age in less than 5% of affected children.
    B.  causes unilateral headache in over 90% of cases.
    C.  when associated with a transient hemiplegia indicates the presence of an underlying brain tumour.
    D.  headaches characteristically have a very sudden onset.
    E.  headaches are usually worse on waking in the morning.

18. **Signs of a 'missed' congenital dislocation of the hip in a 2-year-old include:**
    A.  a positive Ortolani sign.
    B.  reduced hip abduction on the affected side.
    C.  'true' shortening of the leg on the affected side.
    D.  positive Trendelenburg test when standing on the affected side.
    E.  asymmetry of the skin crease of the thigh.

19. **The following conditions are associated with rickets:**
    A.  renal failure.
    B.  prematurity.
    C.  hypothyroidism.
    D.  cystinosis.
    E.  vitamin D receptor insensitivity.

16. **ABC**
'Petit mal' epilepsy is one of the genetic epilepsies characterised by brief loss of awareness, without loss of posture or other associated seizure activity. The EEG shows a typical 3 cycles per second spike and wave pattern which may be brought out by hyperventilating. The episodes may be fleeting. If fits occur frequently, a child's ability to concentrate and learn may be impaired. Treatment is usually with ethosuxamide or sodium valproate.

17. **None of these – all false**
Migraine begins before 10 years in more than 20% of affected children. Headache is unilateral in only 40% of cases – more often frontal or generalised. Migraine is occasionally associated with transient visual, motor or sensory disturbance – with a typical history and with no abnormal physical signs such severe symptoms are very unlikely to be caused by a brain tumour. Explosive onset of migraine headaches is very unusual. Headache worse in the morning, on bending or coughing is suggestive of raised intracranial pressure.

18. **BDE**
The 'clunk' of a dislocated hip relocating within the acetabulum is not felt outside the neonatal period. Abduction of the hip will be restricted on the affected side. The dislocated head of the femur lies above and behind the acetabulum, causing asymmetry of skin creases of the thigh, and results in *apparent* shortening of the affected leg (measure anterior iliac crest to the ankle). True leg length (measure greater trochanter to the ankle) is normal. The gluteal muscles cannot work efficiently – a positive Trendelenburg test results when standing on the affected leg.

19. **ABDE**
In renal failure there is defective hydroxylation of vitamin D to the more active dihydroxycholecalciferol. During the rapid growth of prematurity, without vitamin and mineral supplementation, there is inadequate intake and absorption of calcium and phosphorus for normal mineralisation of bones. Cystinosis is associated with defective proximal renal tubular function, phosphaturia and rickets. In vitamin D resistant rickets there is hypophosphataemia and X-linked dominant inheritance.

20. **Factors associated with a poor prognosis in cystic fibrosis include:**
    A. pancreatic sufficiency.
    B. acquisition of *Burkholderia cepacia.*
    C. meconium ileus.
    D. cor pulmonale.
    E. male sex.

**20. BD**

Pancreatic sufficiency is associated with mild CF disease and a less severe chloride ion channel defect. *B. cepacia*, an invasive pathogen, is associated with a decreased length of survival. With good neonatal surgery and intensive care, meconium ileus is not associated with poor prognosis. Cor pulmonale in cystic fibrosis results from very severe, long-standing lung disease and inevitably has a poor prognosis. The prognosis was better for males than females but, in recent years, this difference has reduced due to increased attention to exercise and fitness in teenaged CF girls.

# 1

# Paediatric surgery

1. **Regarding fluid balance for a newborn infant undergoing surgery:**
   A. there is a lesser ability to excrete a solute load compared with an older child.
   B. the glomerular filtration rate is reduced compared to an older child.
   C. loss of additional 400 ml water due to diarrhoea will not cause a clinically significant problem.
   D. the circulating blood volume will be approximately 600 ml.
   E. three blood-soaked swabs during surgery represent clinically significant blood loss.

2. **Comparing the post-operative requirements of an infant with an adult:**
   A. an infant will require less millilitres of water per kilogram per day than an adult.
   B. an infant will require more mmol of sodium per kilogram per day.
   C. an infant will require fewer grams of protein per kilogram per day.
   D. the adult will require more mmol of iron per kilogram per day.
   E. the adult will require more grams of carbohydrate per kilogram per day.

3. **When examining a swelling in the scrotum of a 4-year-old boy, the following elements are important features:**
   A. the site of the swelling.
   B. the temperature of the swelling.
   C. whether or not there is a cough impulse.
   D. the presence of a bruit by auscultation over the testes.
   E. whether or not lymph nodes at other sites are enlarged.

4. **The following cervical swellings are located in the midline:**
   A. branchial cyst.
   B. sternomastoid tumour.
   C. submental lymph node.
   D. dermoid cyst.
   E. parotid swelling.

1. **ABE**
   It is important to remember that circulating volume and total body water relative to body weight are higher in an infant, while glomerular filtration rate and ability to excrete a solute load are diminished. In the newborn circulating blood volume is approximately 85 ml/kg. Three bloodstained swabs may contain 30 ml blood (around 10% of the circulating volume). Similarly, loss of 'small' volumes of fluid from other sources (vomit, diarrhoea, urine, insensible loss) may be clinically significant.

2. **B**
   Typical requirements of all nutritional elements are higher in infants when expressed in units per kilogram per day. Infants need nutrients for both homeostasis and growth; adults' requirements are predominantly for homeostasis.

3. **ABCDE**
   Examination of swellings in children follows similar principles to adults. Accurate description of the swelling should include: site, size, shape, mobility, temperature, tenderness, colour, consistency, fluctuation, ability to transilluminate, presence of a thrill or bruit (unlikely to be present in this context), regional and generalised lymphadenopathy and the presence of a cough impulse.

4. **CD**
   Branchial cysts appear below the anterior border of the sternomastoid; a sternomastoid tumour occurs within the muscle. Enlarged lymph nodes are generally found laterally but the submental node is located just behind the symphysis of the mandible. Dermoid cysts are usually just below the mandible or suprasternal, along lines of fusion. A thyroglossal cyst is usually found in the midline and moves with protrusion of the tongue. The parotid and submandibular salivary glands are not midline structures.

5. **A child is born with a cavernous haemangioma:**
   A. the parents should be advised the lesion will regress completely within 6 months.
   B. intervention will be needed if there is airway compression.
   C. cosmetics can be used to improve the appearance.
   D. recurrent haemorrhage from trivial trauma is a problem in a minority of cases.
   E. thrombocytopenia may occur.

6. **In a young child with abdominal pain:**
   A. reluctance to play suggests a psychological cause.
   B. vomiting indicates the diagnosis is gastroenteritis.
   C. if the child is lying still, with shallow respirations, it is indicative of colic.
   D. the pain may be due to basal pneumonia.
   E. persistent resistance to palpation makes it likely there is abdominal tenderness.

7. **In appendicitis:**
   A. the pain is typically located in the right iliac fossa at the outset.
   B. a high fever is characteristic.
   C. vomiting is not seen.
   D. rectal tenderness is characteristic of a pelvic appendix.
   E. in some cases, the diagnosis requires laparotomy for confirmation.

8. **In differentiating mesenteric adenitis from appendicitis:**
   A. a history of recent viral respiratory tract infection is typical of mesenteric adenitis.
   B. a low-grade fever makes mesenteric adenitis more likely.
   C. palpable lymph nodes in the abdomen are indicative of appendicitis.
   D. lack of progression of abdominal signs and symptoms is useful in excluding appendicitis.
   E. right iliac fossa pain makes mesenteric adenitis unlikely.

5. **BCDE**

   A cavernous haemangioma is composed of a mass of abnormal blood vessels. The natural history is of enlargement for up to 12 months (sometimes longer) and then to gradually regress over a few years until there is minimal disfigurement. Management is therefore to avoid intervention where possible. Intervention (laser therapy, embolisation, surgery) is considered when the haemangioma is compressing vital structures, or when there is persistent bleeding or a consumptive thrombocytopenia, although intervention is fraught with problems.

6. **DE**

   The clinical characteristics of the acute abdomen in adults can be extended to children but in infants and toddlers the assessment can be more difficult. Observation of the child's behaviour can be as useful as palpation. Lethargy, distress and lack of normal activities are indicative of significant pathology. Vomiting, although non-specific, raises the possibility of a more significant disorder. A child who lies still with shallow breathing may have peritonitis. A child with colic is likely to cry and to draw up the knees intermittently. Extra-abdominal causes should always be considered in the differential diagnosis.

7. **DE**

   The early pain of appendicitis is characteristically diffuse or central with later migration of the pain to the right iliac fossa. If there is a fever, it is low grade; vomiting may occur. Ultrasound examination may provide useful information. In equivocal cases, a decision to perform a laparotomy is often necessary to avoid the hazard of a delayed diagnosis and peritonitis.

8. **AD**

   Mesenteric adenitis is a viral illness, followed by reactive lymphadenopathy in the mesentery. This causes abdominal pain, often with tenderness in the right iliac fossa. Differentiation from appendicitis is based on the association with a viral illness, often with a significant fever; the abdominal signs are more non-specific and lack the typical progression of appendicitis. From the above description, it can be seen that these differences can be subtle and surgical exploration may be necessary in doubtful cases.

9. **Regarding ano-rectal malformations:**
   A. congenital anal stenosis and imperforate anus should be diagnosed soon after birth.
   B. anal dilatation is rarely necessary after corrective surgery.
   C. in imperforate anus at a high level, achieving faecal continence will depend on the pelvic floor muscles.
   D. high-level imperforate anus can usually be treated with a primary correction in the neonatal period.
   E. the prognosis for normal continence after correction of high-level imperforate anus is excellent.

10. **Necrotising enterocolitis:**
    A. usually occurs in previously healthy infants.
    B. often presents with bilious vomiting.
    C. can be diagnosed when bubbles of gas are seen in the bowel wall on an abdominal radiograph.
    D. requires immediate laparotomy to explore the abdomen.
    E. is characteristically associated with noisy, frequent bowel sounds.

11. **Intussusception:**
    A. occurs when a segment of small intestine twists on the mesenteric axis leading to ischaemia of the gut.
    B. most commonly affects school-age children.
    C. is associated with bouts of inconsolable crying.
    D. can be easily diagnosed early in the condition.
    E. can often be treated without surgery.

12. **Posterior urethral valves:**
    A. can be diagnosed antenatally.
    B. may present with ascites.
    C. only affects girls.
    D. are unlikely to affect renal function in the long term.
    E. require urgent surgical treatment.

9. **AC**

Anal stenosis and imperforate anus should be diagnosed soon after birth as a result of neonatal physical examination or abdominal distension with failure of passage of meconium. Congenital anal stenosis is treated by anoplasty but regular anal dilatation will be required for several months after surgery. Imperforate anus is classified into high/intermediate and low types. High/intermediate types are more difficult to treat because of the absence of the external anal sphincter. Continence is therefore dependent on the puborectalis mechanism; however, many children do not achieve good control of continence. A common approach is to perform a colostomy in the neonatal period followed by repair at around 1 year.

10. **BC**

Necrotising enterocolitis typically affects preterm infants, often with other complications of prematurity. Presentation is with abdominal distension and tenderness, vomiting of feeds and blood in the stool. Intramural gas on radiography is diagnostic. There is usually an ileus and an absence of bowel sounds. Management is conservative with parenteral nutrition and antibiotics. Most affected babies will not require surgery. Indications for surgery include perforation, fulminating disease with systemic deterioration and obstruction.

11. **CE**

Intussusception occurs when a segment of bowel 'telescopes' into the lumen of the adjacent bowel lumen leading to obstruction. It typically affects infants between 3 months and 3 years who present with persistent crying. Reduction of the intussusception can often be achieved in the radiology department by air or contrast enema.

12. **ABE**

Posterior urethral valves cause obstruction and distension of the urinary tract from urethra to kidney. Ultrasound scans allow antenatal diagnosis. Extravasation of urine from a hydro-nephrotic kidney may cause ascites. The condition affects only males. After surgery, a degree of renal impairment often persists. Clinical diagnosis can be difficult and contrast studies are usually necessary.

13. **In an infant with oesophageal atresia:**
    A. the diagnosis is suggested by the presence of excess frothy saliva soon after birth.
    B. if there is an 'H-type' fistula, both oesophageal atresia and a tracheo-oesophageal fistula are present.
    C. a contrast swallow is required to establish the presence of the defect.
    D. the presence of air in the stomach excludes the diagnosis of oesophageal atresia.
    E. surgical repair is usually not possible.

14. **In infantile pyloric stenosis:**
    A. the obstruction is due to hypertrophy of the pyloric smooth muscle.
    B. the symptoms typically appear between 4 and 6 months.
    C. the diagnosis may be established by clinical examination.
    D. the infant is likely to be reluctant to feed in the early stages.
    E. vomiting gastric acid leads to a metabolic alkalosis.

15. **In the investigation and treatment of infantile pyloric stenosis:**
    A. surgery should always be performed soon after admission in cases with dehydration.
    B. ultrasound scanning of the abdomen can be used to confirm the diagnosis.
    C. surgical resection of the affected area is the operation of choice.
    D. about 30% of cases can be managed conservatively.
    E. recurrent obstruction in later years is almost unknown.

16. **Duodenal obstruction may be due to:**
    A. duodenal atresia.
    B. an annular pancreas.
    C. Hirschsprung's disease.
    D. an intraluminal diaphragm.
    E. malrotation with intraperitoneal bands.

13.  **A**

Oesophageal atresia and tracheo-oesophageal fistula occur together in a variety of forms. In the commonest variant there is oesophageal atresia and a fistula connecting the trachea to the distal part of the oesophagus, thus permitting passage of air into the gut. The 'H-type' fistula connects the two lumens but there is no oesophageal atresia. Affected infants typically produce large volumes of frothy secretions which may cause cyanosis. The presence of oesophageal atresia can be confirmed by showing that a large-bore orogastric tube cannot pass into the stomach on a plain radiograph. Surgical repair is possible in virtually all cases, although some persistent respiratory or feeding difficulties are common.

14.  **ACE**

Symptoms of this condition typically develop between 4 and 6 weeks of age. The age of onset and characteristic projectile vomiting are suggestive. Examination of the abdomen may reveal visible peristalsis from left to right across the upper abdomen and a palpable mass deep to the right rectus muscle. Affected infants typically feed hungrily, although vomiting; anorexia is a worrying sign of electrolyte disturbance and dehydration. Loss of gastric hydrochloric acid leads to a hypochloraemic metabolic alkalosis.

15.  **BE**

Although the diagnosis is primarily clinical, contrast studies and ultrasound can be helpful if the diagnosis is uncertain. The priority after admission is correction of the dehydration and electrolyte abnormalities prior to surgery. Very few cases will resolve without surgery. The operation of choice is pyloromyotomy (Ramstedt's procedure), which involves incision of the serosa and muscle over the pylorus but leaving the mucosa intact. The operation is highly successful with minimal morbidity and no long-term problems.

16.  **ABDE**

Hirschsprung's disease affects the large bowel beginning at the anus and extending for a variable distance proximally. All other options are recognised causes of duodenal atresia.

17. **In a newborn infant with vomiting, the following features increase the likelihood that the diagnosis is duodenal atresia:**
    A. the absence of bile in the vomit.
    B. generalised abdominal distension.
    C. Down syndrome.
    D. a history of polyhydramnios during the pregnancy.
    E. a 'double bubble' gas shadow on abdominal radiography.

18. **The principles of investigation and treatment of intestinal obstruction in infancy include:**
    A. routine passage of a nasogastric tube to drain the stomach.
    B. early surgery when volvulus is suspected.
    C. administration of intravenous fluids once the urea is greater than 10 mmol/L.
    D. establishing the level of obstruction at laparotomy.
    E. identification of associated malformations once surgery is complete.

19. **Meconium ileus:**
    A. is a form of intestinal obstruction secondary to inspissated bowel contents in the newborn.
    B. is exclusively seen in cystic fibrosis.
    C. may be complicated by peritonitis.
    D. can be relieved by the passage of water-soluble contrast media.
    E. never requires surgical intervention.

20. **The following are presentations of Hirschsprung's disease:**
    A. enterocolitis with diarrhoea.
    B. meconium ileus.
    C. acute obstruction in the neonatal period.
    D. chronic constipation in childhood.
    E. delayed passage of meconium.

17.  **CDE**

Duodenal atresia is associated with polyhydramnios and Down syndrome. Vomit is typically bile stained, although this is a variable finding, depending on whether or not the obstruction is complete and the precise level of obstruction relative to the ampulla of Vater. There may be some distension of the upper abdomen, but this is not a marked feature in upper intestinal obstruction. Gaseous distension of the stomach and duodenum produces a characteristic 'double bubble' on X-ray.

18.  **AB**

In suspected intestinal obstruction the priorities are to resuscitate and stabilise the child, and to establish the level and nature of the obstruction as accurately as possible prior to laparotomy. This is principally achieved with the 'drip and suck' routine: provide intravenous fluids and empty the stomach. Early fluid therapy should prevent dehydration before it develops. Radiological studies defining the level of obstruction greatly improve the chance of successful surgery. Many of the intestinal malformations which cause obstruction are associated with other types of malformation, which may affect the prognosis and postoperative care. To some degree, a volvulus is an exception to these principles because of the risk of gut infarction, sepsis and cardiorespiratory failure secondary to gut ischaemia. However, even in these cases, resuscitation prior to surgery is still vital.

19.  **ACD**

Meconium ileus is associated with cystic fibrosis but also complicates intestinal atresia and stenosis. If the intestine perforates, a chemical peritonitis follows. Where possible, the meconium is cleared by water-soluble contrast enema but in a significant proportion of cases surgical intervention will be necessary.

20.  **ABCDE**

Most cases of Hirschsprung's disease present with acute or subacute obstruction in the neonatal period. Some infants have symptoms from birth in association with meconium ileus. Delayed passage of meconium is extremely common in affected individuals. In less severe cases, presentation may be delayed, causing chronic constipation. Children with Hirschsprung's disease are prone to a particularly severe form of enterocolitis, which may be fatal.

21. **In Hirschsprung's disease:**
    A. there is absence of ganglion cells extending in a patchy distribution through the colon.
    B. there is a familial tendency.
    C. a definitive diagnosis is reached following contrast enema.
    D. resection and primary anastomosis should be achieved in all cases.
    E. there is an association with Down syndrome.

22. **The following conditions cause melaena in childhood:**
    A. anal fissure.
    B. ulcerative colitis.
    C. Meckel's diverticulum.
    D. peptic ulceration.
    E. polyposis coli.

23. **Biliary atresia:**
    A. commonly presents with jaundice within 48 hours of birth.
    B. causes unconjugated hyperbilirubinaemia.
    C. is usually diagnosed by hepatic radioisotope scanning.
    D. has a better prognosis if surgery is deferred until after 1 year.
    E. if untreated, is usually fatal within 2 years.

24. **Exomphalos:**
    A. is a protrusion of abdominal viscera through a defect in the anterior abdominal wall adjacent to the umbilical cord.
    B. is composed of abdominal viscera, amnion and Wharton's jelly.
    C. should be nursed exposed to allow drying of the superficial membranes.
    D. increases the risk of hypothermia in the neonate.
    E. must always be returned to the abdominal cavity within 24 hours of birth.

21. **BE**

In Hirschsprung's disease there a failure of the normal migration of neuroblasts. The point at which migration was interrupted determines the level of the disease. Hirschsprung's is therefore a continuous lesion, starting from the anus and extending a variable distance proximally: 70% of cases affect only the sigmoid and colon; 10% of cases affect the entire colon; and 1–2% affect the small bowel. The risk of an affected sibling is as high as 1 in 10 in those with extensive disease. X-ray features may be suggestive but a rectal biopsy is needed for definitive diagnosis. In some cases, a primary anastomosis is secured, but for many a colostomy is created to relieve the obstruction with the aim of an anastomosis at a later date.

22. **CD**

Melaena follows bleeding in the upper gastrointestinal tract. Bleeding in the lower tract causes blood in the stool. A Meckel's diverticulum is an ectopic piece of gastric mucosa in an appendix-like diverticulum in the ileum which secretes acid and causes ulceration.

23. **CE**

Biliary atresia causes obstruction to biliary drainage, with a gradual rise in conjugated bilirubin. It generally presents late (several days or weeks after birth). This is a significant problem because early operation improves the prospect of achieving effective biliary drainage.

24. **BD**

Exomphalos is a congenital herniation of the abdominal viscera into the umbilical cord. After birth, infants are at risk of hypothermia because of their relatively large surface area and moist exposed hernia sac. The exomphalos is also prone to desiccation and should be protected by polythene wrapping soon after birth. The aim is to return the organs to the abdomen to prevent further complications. In large lesions the hernia is covered by skin flaps alone or by an artificial sac of Silastic and Teflon. In these cases, the sutures are gradually tightened forcing the abdominal cavity to accommodate the organs and finally permitting closure.

**25. An infant with gastroschisis:**
  A. has a sac enclosing the protruding bowel.
  B. has a high likelihood of having other congenital abnormalities.
  C. is likely to become hypoproteinaemic.
  D. is likely to have enteral feeding fully established within 3 days of surgical closure.
  E. should have a nasogastric tube passed immediately after birth.

**26. Prune belly syndrome:**
  A. is associated with failure of development of the anterior abdominal wall muscles.
  B. is usually associated with dilatation of the urinary tract.
  C. is commonly associated with cryptorchidism.
  D. requires radiological assessment of the urinary tract soon after birth.
  E. is twice as common in girls than boys.

**27. Hypospadias:**
  A. is often associated with defective development of tissue on the ventral surface causing downward angulation of the penis.
  B. is the opening of the urinary meatus on the dorsal surface of the penis.
  C. is an indication for early circumcision.
  D. is found in 1 in 5000 male infants.
  E. requires surgical correction if there is misdirection of the urinary stream.

**28. A mother brings her 4-month-old son to out-patients reporting an intermittent swelling in the scrotum:**
  A. if it is not possible to palpate above the mass, the diagnosis of inguinal hernia is likely.
  B. a hernia is most easily seen with the child lying supine.
  C. if no swelling is found, the mother's observations can be safely discounted.
  D. if an inguinal hernia is diagnosed, it should be repaired electively around the age of 2 years.
  E. there is more likely to be an inguinal hernia if the child was born prematurely.

**25.    CE**

Gastroschisis is a congenital defect involving herniation of the gut. In contrast to exomphalos, the gut herniates through an abdominal wall defect lateral to the umbilicus, is not protected by a sac and is rarely associated with other congenital abnormalities. It is common for intestinal function to take several weeks to recover after closure of the defect. Parenteral nutrition is of vital importance in the postoperative care of these infants. Bowel dysfunction may result from low-grade injury due to exposure and congestion at the orifice of the hernia. The nasogastric tube is passed to minimise bowel distension. Hypoproteinaemia can occur by exudation from the bowel.

**26.    ABCD**

Prune belly syndrome comprises failure of development of anterior abdominal wall musculature, urinary tract dilatation with hydronephrosis, bilateral cryptorchidism and urinary meatal stenosis. It is mostly found in boys.

**27.    AE**

Hypospadias is the abnormal location of the urinary meatus on the ventral surface of the penis, often associated with deficient tissue on the inferior surface causing downwards angulation of the penis, termed chordee. Indications for correction include meatal stenosis, chordee and marked displacement of the urinary stream. The foreskin may be employed in the repair and circumcision is contraindicated. The defect is common affecting around 1 in 160 male infants.

**28.    AE**

An inguinal hernia descends from the abdomen towards the scrotum; it is impossible to palpate an upper limit. By contrast, in a hydrocele fluid collects in the fundus of the processus vaginalis. Smaller hernias fluctuate in size and are more likely to be evident if the child is held upright. On occasions, no sign of the hernia will be present at the time of examination, but if the parent's description is clear, one should arrange a further examination at a later date or even consider surgical explora-tion. The hernia may strangulate, so repair is performed at the earliest available date. Preterm infants are more likely to develop hernias.

**29. A newborn boy is examined and neither testis can be found in the scrotum:**
   A. there is a 10% chance that the testes will spontaneously descend before 12 months of age.
   B. surgery is indicated if the testes remain undescended at 2 years of age.
   C. if the testes are undescended, there is an increased risk of malignant change.
   D. persistent undescended testes are associated with normal fertility.
   E. the undescended testis cannot undergo torsion.

**30. In the management of lip and palate defects:**
   A. the parents of a baby with isolated cleft lip should be advised that normal breast feeding should be possible.
   B. a thorough examination should be conducted for other malformations.
   C. the risk of a further affected infant in the same family is negligible.
   D. there is an increased risk of hearing impairment in later years.
   E. routine adenoidectomy is indicated at the time of repair of cleft palate.

**29. BC**

About 3% of newborns have undescended testes but around two-thirds of these will spontaneously descend during the first year. Undescended testes require surgical intervention to improve the prospect of fertility, to reduce the risk of torsion or trauma and because of the risk of malignancy. It is not clear whether or not orchidopexy reduces the risk of malignant change, but at least it places the testis in a location where it can be easily examined. Severely dysplastic testes are generally removed.

**30. ABD**

Cleft lip does not affect normal feeding, unlike cleft palate. There is an increased risk of further affected children in the same family but there is not a simple pattern of Mendelian inheritance. Most children with cleft lip or palate are otherwise normal but these lesions are elements of many syndromes involving multiple malformations. There is an increased risk of speech difficulty because of palatal dysfunction and of hearing impairment from serous otitis media, which is common. Following palatal repair, there is a risk of nasal air escape during speech; adenoidectomy is therefore contraindicated in children with cleft palate.

# 2

## Respiratory

1. **Regarding respiratory tract infections:**
   A. a normal preschool child may have up to ten upper respiratory tract infections in a single year.
   B. half of the respiratory tract infections occurring in early childhood involve the lower respiratory tract.
   C. simple nasal obstruction will cause feeding difficulty in infants.
   D. the commonest infecting agent causing the common cold is the rhinovirus.
   E. Streptococcal pharyngitis can be diagnosed on clinical grounds with confidence.

2. **The following organisms commonly cause community acquired respiratory tract infection:**
   A. respiratory syncytial virus.
   B. *Streptococcus pneumoniae.*
   C. *Pneumocystis carinii.*
   D. *Pseudomonas aeruginosa.*
   E. parainfluenza virus.

3. **In croup:**
   A. stridor typically develops 1–2 days after the onset of coryzal symptoms.
   B. stridor is predominantly expiratory in the early stages.
   C. irritability should be relieved by mild sedation.
   D. antibiotic therapy will reduce the duration of the illness.
   E. nebulised adrenaline will reduce the severity of airflow obstruction

4. **In epiglottitis:**
   A. *Haemophilus influenza* type B is usually isolated from blood cultures.
   B. a temperature above 38.5°C would cast doubt on the diagnosis.
   C. children characteristically prefer to sit straight upright.
   D. virtually all cases will require endotracheal intubation.
   E. an intramuscular dose of an appropriate antibiotic should be given as early as possible before the child reaches hospital.

1. **ACD**

   The average preschool child has between eight and twelve respiratory infections in 1 year. Most are confined to the upper respiratory tract. Infants breathe predominantly through the nose and nasal obstruction from the common cold can make feeding exceedingly difficult. Over 90% of respiratory infections are due to viruses but these are difficult to distinguish clinically from bacterial infections.

2. **ABE**

   Respiratory tract infections are commonly caused by viruses (rhinovirus, respiratory syncytial virus, parainfluenza, influenza and adenovirus) and less frequently by bacteria (*Streptococcus pneumoniae, Beta-haemolytic streptococcus, Haemophilus influenzae* and *Mycoplasma pneumoniae*). Infections with organisms of low pathogenicity, such as *Pneumocystis carinii* or *Pseudomonas aeruginosa*, should raise the possibility of an abnormal predisposition to infection such as cystic fibrosis or an immunodeficiency.

3. **AE**

   In croup (laryngo-tracheo-bronchitis) there is commonly a prodromal coryzal illness for 1–2 days before stridor develops. In epiglottitis stridor often develops within hours of the onset of the illness. Stridor is predominantly an inspiratory noise; an expiratory noise suggests more severe airway obstruction. Croup is usually caused by parainfluenza virus but also by rhinovirus, influenza and respiratory syncytial virus infections. Antibiotics are not indicated. Nebulised adrenaline relieves airway obstruction, probably by reducing laryngeal and subglottic mucosal oedema. Sedation should be avoided.

4. **ACD**

   Epiglottitis is caused by *Haemophilus influenza* type B. Affected children are often septicaemic with a high fever, lethargy and look 'toxic' (unlike children with croup). The child will usually prefer to sit up and be unable to swallow their secretions. In epiglottitis virtually all cases will require endotracheal intubation until the swelling resolves. As distressing the child may precipitate complete airway obstruction, manoeuvres such as venepuncture and inspection of the throat should be deferred until after intubation by an experienced anaesthetist.

5. **In a child with symptoms characteristic of whooping cough:**
   A. a lymphocyte count of 24.7 × $10^9$ per litre in the peripheral blood film supports the diagnosis of pertussis infection.
   B. the symptoms might be caused by adenovirus.
   C. erythromycin will completely resolve symptoms within 10 days.
   D. persistence of cough for more than 6 weeks suggests the diagnosis is other than whooping cough.
   E. the risk of brain damage is higher if the child is under 1 year old.

6. **The following are recognised complications of whooping cough:**
   A. epistaxis.
   B. apnoea.
   C. subconjunctival haemorrhage.
   D. weight loss.
   E. cyanotic attacks.

7. **A previously well 3-year-old child is taken to his general practitioner with a 2-day history of coryzal symptoms and a 1-day history of cough productive of sputum. Physical examination reveals rhinorrhoea and a low-grade fever, but no other abnormalities and the chest is clear:**
   A. the presence of cough following viral infection makes the diagnosis of asthma likely.
   B. the presence of cough indicates lower respiratory tract involvement.
   C. the production of sputum implies secondary bacterial infection.
   D. an expectorant cough mixture will be helpful in ameliorating the symptoms.
   E. the commonest cause of these symptoms would be viral bronchitis.

8. **The following findings are suggestive of bronchiolitis:**
   A. expiratory wheezing and inspiratory crackles heard on chest auscultation.
   B. fever of 39.5°C.
   C. hyperinflation of the chest.
   D. widespread patchy opacification of the lung fields on a chest radiograph.
   E. identification of respiratory syncytial virus in nasopharyngeal secretions.

5.  **ABE**

    An absolute lymphocytosis is characteristic of the prodromal phase of *Bordetella pertussis* infection. A whooping cough-like illness may be caused by *B. pertussis, B. parapertussis* and adenovirus. Erythromycin given early in the illness reduces the period of infectivity but has no significant impact on the illness itself. The paroxysmal cough typically persists for up to 8 weeks and some patients continue with some degree of cough for up to 6 months. Complications of pneumonia, encephalopathy and death are all commoner in infants.

6.  **ABCDE – all of these**

    In whooping cough a tracheobronchitis causes paroxysmal bouts of coughing, sometimes climaxing in an inspiratory whoop. Complications are commoner in infancy, particularly under 3 months of age. The coughing spasms may cause vomiting and weight loss. Venous congestion of the head and neck may produce subconjunctival haemorrhage and epistaxis. Young infants may become apnoeic.

7.  **BE**

    Most community acquired respiratory tract infections mainly affect the upper respiratory tract. Viral bronchitis is common and may result in sputum production (which does not necessarily signify bacterial infection). There is no evidence that 'expectorant' drugs are effective. The presence of a cough implies that the infection has involved the larynx, trachea or bronchial tree (the lower respiratory tract). A previous history of recurrent cough or wheeze with viral infections would suggest a diagnosis of asthma but neither is present here.

8.  **ACE**

    Respiratory syncytial virus antigen can be identified using a fluorescent antibody technique on the nasopharyngeal secretions. There is a low-grade fever. Bronchiolitis causes inflammation of bronchioles which results in hyperinflation of the chest. Wheezing is caused by turbulent airflow in large airways which are narrowed during expiration. Inspiratory crackles are due to secretions and to the opening of small airways which are occluded in expiration. The chest radiograph may show hyperinflation, peribronchial thickening and, in some cases, segmental or lobar collapse. Patchy opacification is more suggestive of bronchopneumonia.

9. **In an infant affected by bronchiolitis:**
   A. broad-spectrum antibiotics should be prescribed immediately.
   B. an oxygen saturation of 85% indicates a need for oxygen therapy.
   C. cough is unlikely to be a prominent symptom.
   D. downwards displacement of the liver edge is indicative of heart failure.
   E. feeding via nasogastric tube may avoid the need for intravenous fluids.

10. **The following features would be consistent with a diagnosis of *Mycoplasma pneumoniae* infection:**
    A. non-specific flu-like symptoms 10 days previously.
    B. similar symptoms in several classmates.
    C. inspiratory crackles on auscultation of the chest.
    D. the identification of cold agglutinins in the bloodstream.
    E. extensive lower lobe infiltrates on the chest radiograph.

11. **The following disorders cause cough as a prominent symptom:**
    A. hay fever.
    B. asthma.
    C. pneumonia.
    D. pharyngitis.
    E. inhaled foreign body.

12. **Stridor is characteristic of:**
    A. bronchiolitis.
    B. laryngo-tracheo-bronchitis (croup).
    C. asthma.
    D. bronchopneumonia.
    E. laryngomalacia.

9.  **BE**

Bronchiolitis is caused by viral infection, most commonly by respiratory syncytial virus. Affected infants usually have a history of initial coryzal symptoms followed by lower respiratory tract symptoms of cough, wheeze and breathlessness. Treatment is supportive, aimed at maintaining fluid intake via nasogastric tube or intravenous infusion and preventing hypoxia. Hypoxia is indicated by an oxygen saturation below the low 90s per cent (normal >96%). Bronchiolar inflammation causes airway narrowing and air trapping which, in turn, produces hyper-inflation of the lungs and downwards displacement of the liver. Heart failure does not occur unless there is pre-existing heart disease.

10. **ABCDE**

*Mycoplasma pneumoniae* is a common cause of pneumonia in school-age children; it is often spread through schools and within families. There is often a prolonged prodromal illness for up to 3 weeks before specific respiratory symptoms develop. Affected individuals are usually not particularly unwell despite abnormalities on clinical and radiological examination of the chest.

11. **BCE**

Cough is caused by mechanical irritation or inflammation of the larynx, trachea, bronchi and bronchioles. Infection or allergy confined to the upper respiratory tract does not cause cough. An inhaled foreign body persistently stimulates cough receptors and should be considered as a possible diagnosis in all children with unexplained chronic cough.

12. **BE**

Stridor is an inspiratory noise caused by obstruction to the extrathoracic airway, most commonly in the larynx. Acute causes of stridor include croup, epiglottitis, an inhaled foreign body in the extrathoracic airway, measles, angioneurotic oedema, retropharyngeal abscess and diphtheria. Chronic stridor may be caused by laryngomalacia, subglottic stenosis after prolonged endotracheal intubation, laryngeal web, papilloma or haemangioma, vocal cord paralysis and malformations of the larynx and trachea such as laryngeal cleft.

13. **Wheezing may be found in children affected by:**
    A. inhaled foreign body.
    B. aspiration of gastric contents.
    C. viral bronchiolitis.
    D. bronchopulmonary dysplasia.
    E. tracheal stenosis.

14. **The following findings are suggestive of a diagnosis of asthma:**
    A. a peak flow diary showing repeated fluctuation between 300 L/min in the evening and 250 L/min in the morning.
    B. a history of recurrent cough after coryzal illnesses.
    C. a drop in peak expiratory flow rate of 14% during an exercise test.
    D. a positive skin test to house dust mite.
    E. a history of failure to thrive during infancy and early childhood.

15. **The following findings make a diagnosis of asthma unlikely:**
    A. lobar collapse identified on a chest radiograph.
    B. cough only occurring during vigorous exercise.
    C. the absence of a family history of asthma.
    D. failure to improve after 2 weeks on high-dose oral steroids.
    E. a cough productive of sputum.

16. **In the treatment of asthma:**
    A. most children over 6 years of age can use a metered-dose aerosol effectively without a spacer.
    B. the use of regular inhaled steroid is limited by a high incidence of side-effects.
    C. advice should be given to restrict the asthmatic child's participation in sport.
    D. oral corticosteroids should be reserved only for children who require hospital admission.
    E. regular anti-inflammatory treatment should be recommended for a child who requires bronchodilator most days.

**13.  ABCDE**

Wheeze is an expiratory noise caused by turbulent airflow and is suggestive of intrathoracic airway obstruction. Wheeze may be due to narrowing at a single site (inhaled foreign body, tracheal stenosis, mediastinal mass, vascular malformation) or generalised airway narrowing (asthma, bronchiolitis, Mycoplasma pneumonia, aspiration of gastric contents, bronchopulmonary dysplasia).

**14.  ABC**

In normal individuals peak flow rate does not fluctuate by more than 10% either with diurnal variation or with exercise. Viral infections occasionally cause cough, but a history of persistent cough in association with coryzal symptoms should raise the possibility of a diagnosis of asthma. Although allergy to house dust mite may exacerbate asthma, a positive skin test suggests an atopic tendency which may not necessarily manifest itself as asthma. Failure to thrive is only rarely seen when asthma is severe.

**15.  D**

A central component of asthma is airway inflammation, and if there is no improvement with oral corticosteroids, the diagnosis should be reconsidered. The inflammation causes hypersecretion of mucus which may lead to lobar collapse by mucus plugging or a productive cough. Although a family history of asthma or atopic illnesses is common in children with asthma, it is not necessary for the diagnosis. Some children's symptoms are exclusively induced by exercise.

**16.  E**

Frequent bronchodilator use suggests chronic active asthma for which anti-inflammatory treatment would be appropriate. Children (and many adults!) have difficulty with the coordination required to use metered dose inhalers effectively. Asthmatic children are best treated with inhaled drug delivered via a spacer device or dry powder inhaler. The aim of therapy should be to control symptoms to permit a normal life, including participation in sport. Oral corticosteroids are useful in controlling chronic symptoms refractory to inhaled therapy, or in preventing deterioration which would be likely to lead to hospital admission.

17. **In acute asthma:**
    A. only bronchodilator given via nebuliser will relieve breathlessness.
    B. children who require hospital admission should receive oral steroids.
    C. a peak flow of 30% of a patient's best value is an indication for admission.
    D. children may be safely managed at home with nebulised bronchodilator given regularly but not more often than at hourly intervals.
    E. pulse oximetry is helpful in evaluating the severity of the attack.

18. **The following drugs can be expected to have a bronchodilator effect within 1 hour of administration:**
    A. budesonide.
    B. aminophylline.
    C. terbutaline.
    D. hydrocortisone.
    E. adrenaline.

19. **The following statements are correct regarding asthma treatment:**
    A. oral salbutamol is comparable in efficacy to inhaled salbutamol.
    B. sodium cromoglycate blocks mast cell degranulation.
    C. inhaled steroid therapy may be effective in controlling asthma in children where sodium cromoglycate has failed.
    D. approximately 10% of children with asthma require long-term oral corticosteroid to achieve satisfactory control.
    E. Salmeterol is a long-acting beta-2 agonist.

20. **A 3-year-old boy is brought to hospital after choking while eating peanuts. He was wheezy for a few minutes but is now asymptomatic:**
    A. the presence of a unilateral wheeze on auscultation would support a diagnosis of an inhaled foreign body.
    B. a chest X-ray is not indicated because a peanut is not radio-opaque.
    C. if he remains asymptomatic for 24 hours and physical examination is normal, he may be safely discharged home without further investigation.
    D. bronchoscopy should be performed as soon as possible.
    E. the risk of lung damage is less because the inhaled material is organic.

**17.   BCE**

In acute asthma larger than usual doses of bronchodilator given using the patient's usual inhaler device may be effective. Parents must be educated to seek medical attention if nebulised bronchodilator need be repeated more often than 4 hourly. A peak flow rate below 50% of predicted after bronchodilator is an indication to seek medical help and a further reduction to less than 30% suggests hospital treatment will be required. Oxygen saturation below 93% suggests a probable need for hospital admission. If admission is required, oral corticosteroids should be prescribed to suppress inflammation and resolve the attack rapidly.

**18.   BCE**

Adrenergic agonists, including beta-2 agonists (salbutamol and terbutaline) are effective, rapid-acting bronchodilators, particularly when administered by the inhaled route. Adrenaline is also an effective drug in acute asthma but generally has been superseded by the more selective beta-2 agonists. Theophylline and aminophylline also have bronchodilator effects but have to be given by the oral or intravenous route. Corticosteroids relieve airway obstruction by suppressing inflammation and take several hours before the effect is clinically apparent.

**19.   BCE**

Inhaled therapy is generally more effective in controlling asthma than oral drugs. A proportion of children with chronic asthma have symptoms which are not effectively controlled by sodium cromoglycate and, in many of these cases, inhaled steroids will be effective. Only a tiny minority (< 1%) of children with asthma require long-term oral corticosteroid to control their symptoms, although many will need occasional short courses to treat acute episodes.

**20.   AD**

The history is highly suggestive of an inhaled foreign body. A bronchoscopy should be performed as soon as possible. Organic material may stimulate an especially marked inflammatory reaction resulting in permanent damage. A unilateral or localised persistent wheeze is supportive of the diagnosis. Organic material is radiolucent but a chest radiograph may show an area of collapse or hyperinflation.

21. **In cystic fibrosis the following organisms chronically colonise the lower respiratory tract:**
    A. *Staphylococcus aureus.*
    B. *Streptococcus pneumoniae.*
    C. *Aspergillus fumigatus.*
    D. *Pseudomonas aeruginosa.*
    E. *Mycoplasma pneumoniae.*

22. **A 10-month-old child is diagnosed as having cystic fibrosis. The parents should be given the following information:**
    A. the child is unlikely to survive into the second decade.
    B. chest physiotherapy occasionally may be needed when there are symptoms of a chest infection.
    C. virtually all children with cystic fibrosis will require pancreatic enzyme supplementation.
    D. there is a 1 in 4 risk of further children being affected by cystic fibrosis.
    E. in hot weather additional salt will be needed.

23. **In cystic fibrosis:**
    A. rectal prolapse may occur in infancy.
    B. distal intestinal obstruction syndrome usually requires surgical intervention.
    C. progressive pancreatic disease may ultimately result in diabetes mellitus.
    D. some patients develop progressive liver disease, which may be fatal.
    E. virtually all females are infertile.

24. **The following conditions will produce obstructive changes in pulmonary function tests:**
    A. asthma.
    B. cystic fibrosis.
    C. fibrosing alveolitis.
    D. muscular dystrophy.
    E. tracheomalacia.

21. **ACD**

In cystic fibrosis impaired mucociliary clearance permits chronic bacterial colonisation of the lower respiratory tract. *Staphylococcus aureus* is usually the earliest pathogen and by adulthood *Pseudomonas aeruginosa* is the commonest infecting organism (70–80% colonised). Colonisation with *Aspergillus fumigatus* may cause an allergic bronchopulmonary aspergillosis. *Streptococcus pneumoniae* and *Mycoplasma pneumoniae* may cause acute infection in cystic fibrosis, but do not generally cause chronic infection.

22. **CDE**

Cystic fibrosis (CF) is autosomal recessive and there is a 1 in 4 risk of carrier parents producing affected children. Pulmonary infection and airway obstruction are treated with regular postural drainage and chest physiotherapy. Pancreatic enzyme supplementation is required by 85% of CF patients. Affected individuals lose large amounts of salt in their sweat and require oral salt supplements in hot weather. The majority of patients today survive into their twenties (mean survival is now 30 years) and the prognosis continues to improve.

23. **ACD**

Rectal prolapse is a complication of cystic fibrosis. Intestinal obstruction may occur as a result of meconium ileus equivalent, now called distal intestinal obstruction syndrome (DIOS). Most cases can be relieved by the use of water contrast media or bowel washout. Diabetes mellitus occurs, with increasing frequency, with age. Clinically significant liver disease affects less than 5% of individuals with cystic fibrosis. Virtually all males are sterile.

24. **ABE**

Obstructive defects are characterised by reduced PEFR, FEV1 and FEV1/FVC ratio. Asthma causes airway obstruction due to mucosal oedema, hypersecretion and bronchospasm. Cystic fibrosis causes thick, viscid secretions, with secondary airway inflammation and infection. Tracheomalacia is a condition in which the cartilage rings in the large airways are deficient leading to airway collapse. Neuromuscular disorders, thoracic skeletal abnormalities and pulmonary fibrosis cause restrictive changes.

**25.** **A 6-year-old boy presents in A&E with persistent productive cough and weight loss. He lives in a hostel for homeless families with his mother, who has just been diagnosed as having pulmonary TB:**
   **A.** a positive tuberculin test confirms a diagnosis of tuberculosis.
   **B.** a negative tuberculin test excludes a diagnosis of tuberculosis.
   **C.** treatment for his asymptomatic brother may be necessary if there is a positive tuberculin test, even if the chest radiograph is normal.
   **D.** the child can be admitted to an open ward because the risk of spread of tuberculosis is very low.
   **E.** other residents in the hostel should have CXR and tuberculin tests.

**26.** **Lung development (structural and functional):**
   **A.** is structurally completed by 34 weeks' gestation.
   **B.** is functionally sufficiently advanced to support gas exchange from 18 weeks' gestation.
   **C.** is dependent on adequate fetal breathing.
   **D.** is structurally accelerated by administration of steroids to the mother.
   **E.** is adversely affected by maternal smoking in pregnancy.

**27.** **In a child with a lower respiratory tract infection:**
   **A.** adenovirus infection may cause a necrotising bronchiolitis.
   **B.** erythema multiforme indicates a likely Mycoplasma infection.
   **C.** chest X-ray consolidation is diagnostic of bacterial infection.
   **D.** pleural fluid seen on X-ray in association with a lower lobe consolidation should be left to resolve with antibiotics.
   **E.** a Mantoux test should always be performed.

**25.  CE**

The tuberculin test detects cell-mediated immune response to tuberculo-protein. In a clinically suspected case, a positive result is supportive evidence but false-positives may occur. False-negatives also occur in some situations. If there is a strong suspicion of TB, treatment is indicated even if the chest radiograph is normal. There is risk of transmission as long as the patient is producing sputum which may contain tubercle. Tuberculosis is commonly spread among individuals living in socially deprived conditions.

**26.  CE**

Lung development is not complete at term. Alveoli continue to develop and mature after birth. The alveoli and pulmonary capillary beds are not sufficiently developed for adequate gas exchange until 23–24 weeks' gestation. Fetal breathing is necessary for normal lung growth. Maternal steroid administration in pregnancy induces surfactant production, but does not affect lung structure. Infants of mothers who smoke in pregnancy have increased airways resistance due to reduced airway calibre.

**27.  AB**

Some serotypes of adenovirus (types 3, 7 & 21) may be associated with destructive lung disease. Erythema multiforme is associated with Herpes and Mycoplasma infections. Radiology cannot distinguish a viral or bacterial cause. An effusion in association with consolidation should be tapped as an empyema (pus in the pleural cavity) needs to be drained. In the UK a Mantoux test is not part of routine investigation of a simple chest infection unless there is a history of TB contact, suggestive X-ray appearance or failure of resolution.

28. **Clinical signs:**
    A. bronchial breathing in the 5th right intercostal space in the subscapular region indicates a right middle lobe pneumonia.
    B. a persistent wheeze with reduced breath sounds is diagnostic of asthma.
    C. a respiratory rate of 40/min is normal for a 5-year-old at rest.
    D. pectus excavatum is a sign of undertreated asthma.
    E. reduced right-sided breath sounds, dullness to percussion and shift of the apex beat to the right are all consistent with a right pleural effusion.

29. **Normal development of the lung in utero:**
    A. is anatomically complete by 36 weeks' gestation.
    B. is complete with regard to development of the airways by 24 weeks' gestation.
    C. is dependent on fetal breathing movements.
    D. proceeds with the lungs partially inflated with amniotic fluid.
    E. will permit satisfactory gas exchange from 18 weeks' gestation.

30. **Lung hypoplasia:**
    A. usually results in intrauterine death.
    B. is present in more than 50% of premature babies requiring ventilation.
    C. will occur in the event of significant fetal muscle weakness.
    D. will occur if there is complete obstruction of the fetal urinary tract.
    E. is caused by maternal malnutrition in pregnancy.

31. **Deviation of the mediastinum to the *right* is caused by:**
    A. a left pleural effusion.
    B. cardiomegaly.
    C. congenital right middle lobe emphysema.
    D. a hypoplastic right lung.
    E. right lower lobe consolidation.

**28. All false**

The surface projection of the right middle lobe lies over the 5th and 6th intercostal space anteriorly. A wheeze only indicates turbulent airflow. A normal respiratory rate for a 5-year-old at rest would be 20–25 breaths/min. The physical signs outlined in question E indicate the presence of right-sided collapse. With a right-sided effusion, deviation of the mediastinum to the left would be expected unless associated with an underlying collapse.

**29. BC**

Development of the conducting airways is complete by 18 weeks. Development of the respiratory bronchioles down to primitive alveolar sacs is complete by 24 weeks' gestation, and it is at this stage that life becomes possible outside the uterus. Normal growth of the fetal lung is dependent on satisfactory breathing movements. Lung fluid is secreted by the airway epithelium and is biochemically different from amniotic fluid.

**30. CD**

Lung hypoplasia will occur if there is an absence of fetal breathing due to neuromuscular disease, or if there is chest compression in the absence of an adequate amniotic fluid volume (including major renal abnormalities) or if there is inadequate space for a lung to develop as with a diaphragmatic hernia. Lung hypoplasia is not critical in fetal life as the placenta provides oxygenation. A small percentage of those premature babies who require ventilation are thought to have a degree of lung hypoplasia. This group is over-represented in autopsy series.

**31. AD**

A pleural effusion will cause mediastinal shift unless associated with an underlying collapse of the lung on the same side. Cardiomegaly does not cause displacement of the mediastinum, but may cause displacement of the apex beat. A congenital right middle lobar emphysema will cause the mediastinum to be displaced to the left. Collapse or hypoplasia of the right lung will cause shift of the mediastinum to the right, but a consolidation of the right lower lobe without loss of volume will cause no mediastinal shift.

32. **Respiratory distress is commoner in young infants than older children and adults because:**
    A. airflow in a bronchus is inversely proportional to the radius of the bronchus.
    B. the chest wall has increased compliance.
    C. an infant's large airways tend to collapse if expiratory effort is increased.
    D. infants are immunodeficient.
    E. there is ventilation and perfusion mismatching.

33. **The arterial blood gas results of a 13-year-old boy breathing room air are as follows: pH 7.32, $PCO_2$ 7.3 Kpa (4.5–6 Kpa), $PO_2$ 6.3 Kpa (10–13 Kpa), Base excess +7 mmol/L (+4 to –4 mmol/L), Standard bicarbonate 30 mmol/L. These results:**
    A. show a respiratory alkalosis.
    B. indicate a primary metabolic abnormality.
    C. are consistent with a recent cardiac arrest.
    D. are consistent with end-stage cystic fibrosis.
    E. are consistent with mild asthma.

34. **With regard to oxygen therapy and monitoring:**
    A. administration of more than 35% oxygen to a child with acute severe asthma will risk precipitating respiratory failure.
    B. 100% oxygen administered to a premature baby with idiopathic respiratory distress syndrome for more than 48 hours will cause retinopathy of prematurity.
    C. inspired oxygen concentration >60% is toxic to type 1 pneumatocytes.
    D. the $PaO_2$ can be accurately predicted from the oxygen dissociation curve for any given level of oxygen saturation.
    E. 30–40% oxygen should be routinely administered to children with croup.

35. **Surfactant:**
    A. increases lung compliance.
    B. is detectable in amniotic fluid.
    C. is produced by the type 2 pneumatocytes.
    D. production is inhibited by any stress affecting the fetus.
    E. is not produced by fetal lungs until after 32 weeks' gestation.

**32.  BCE**

Airflow in tubes is directly proportional to the fourth power of the radius. The soft chest wall makes inspiratory efforts less effective due to sternal and costal recession. Increased compliance of the large airways causes them also to collapse during active expiration. Although infants are not strictly immunodeficient, they are immunologically inexperienced and need to build up their own immunity to infections once maternal antibody levels have waned. There is an exaggerated ventilation–perfusion mismatch at both extremes of life.

**33.  D**

These results show a compensated respiratory acidosis with a moderate degree of hypoxaemia. There is a reduced pH, indicating a mild *acidosis* (pH less than 7.4). The raised $CO_2$ indicates a respiratory acidosis, and the raised standard bicarbonate level indicates that there has been a metabolic compensation for the respiratory acidosis, and that this is not an acute problem. After cardiac arrest or marked exertion, there is an accumulation of lactic acid causing a base deficit.

**34.  C**

Loss of $CO_2$ responsiveness very rarely occurs in paediatric medicine except in children affected by severe cystic fibrosis and muscle disorders. In general, it is appropriate to give sufficient oxygen to prevent hypoxia. Hyperoxaemia is one of the risk factors for retinopathy of prematurity, but high inspired oxygen concentrations can be used with careful monitoring of $PaO_2$. Inspired $O_2$ concentration > 50% is toxic to respiratory epithelium. The $PaO_2$ cannot be predicted from the $SaO_2$ as environmental conditions may shift the oxygen dissociation curve to left or right. Children with croup require only oxygen when they have severe airway obstruction and therefore it is not routinely administered.

**35.  ABC**

Surfactant is produced by the type 2 pneumatocytes of the respiratory epithelium. Over the last trimester of pregnancy, surfactant is produced in increasing amounts in preparation for birth. Fetal stress increases fetal cortisol output leading to increased surfactant production. Surfactant can be detected and measured in amniotic fluid. At delivery, surfactant acts to reduce the surface tension forces tending to collapse the airspaces and so reduces the stiffness of the lung – i.e. increases compliance.

36. **In a 3-year-old boy an inhaled foreign body:**
    A. can be seen on chest X-ray in over 70% of affected cases.
    B. should be suspected if there is persistent overinflation of a lobe.
    C. should be suspected if there is persistent collapse of a lobe.
    D. should be suspected if there is wheeze responsive to beta-2 agonists.
    E. should be treated conservatively with antibiotics and physiotherapy.

37. **Recurrent aspiration pneumonia:**
    A. is associated with fat-laden macrophages in the sputum.
    B. is associated with cerebral palsy.
    C. causes predominantly left upper lobe consolidation.
    D. can be diagnosed with an isotope milk scan.
    E. is caused by an 'H-type' tracheo-oesophageal fistula.

38. **In bronchopulmonary dysplasia:**
    A. only preterm ventilated babies are affected.
    B. calorie requirement is normal.
    C. there is a very short expiratory time.
    D. there is hyperinflation of the chest.
    E. there is inevitable progression of the disease to cor pulmonale in the majority of affected babies.

**36. BC**

In young children an inhaled foreign body should be suspected if there are localised respiratory signs or radiological abnormalities which do not resolve. Inhaled foreign bodies (e.g. peanuts or plastic) are usually radiolucent and cannot be seen on X-ray. Whenever a foreign body is suspected from the history, examination or radiological findings, then bronchoscopy is mandatory.

**37. ABDE**

Alveolar macrophages will ingest fat that has been aspirated into the lungs. Positive Sudan Red staining of secretions from the lower respiratory tract after bronchial lavage (for fat) may suggest the diagnosis. Technetium isotope may be added to a feed and the lungs scanned sometime after feeding. If isotope is found within the lungs, then this is diagnostic of aspiration. Children with cerebral palsy are at increased risk of aspiration pneumonias, particularly if they have swallowing difficulties, gastro-oesophageal reflux or a hiatus hernia. Aspiration pneumonia typically affects the right lung, but can involve the whole lung. 'H-type' tracheo-oesophageal fistulas will cause recurrent soiling of the lungs with oesphageal or gastric contents – the right upper lobe tends to be the most severely affected.

**38. D**

Bronchopulmonary dysplasia or chronic lung disease of prematurity mainly but not exclusively affects *ventilated* infants. Increased respiratory effort causes a very significant increase in calorie requirement for normal growth, which may be difficult to match. The respiratory disease is characterised by air trapping in a hyperinflated chest with a prolonged expiratory phase often accompanied by wheezing. There may be some response to bronchodilators or anticholinergic agents. With adequate respiratory support and attention to ensuring adequate oxygenation, most babies will recover from their chronic lung disease over time with growth and development of the lungs.

# 3

# Neonatology

1. **The following are accepted definitions:**
   A. the *neonatal* period is the first 28 days of life of a newborn of any gestation.
   B. *small for gestation* infants have a birthweight less than the 10th centile.
   C. *infancy* refers to the 1st year of life.
   D. the *neonatal mortality rate* is the number of deaths in the first 28 days per 1000 live births.
   E. the *fetal period* is from the 12th week of gestation to delivery.

2. **The Apgar score:**
   A. is only measured in asphyxiated babies.
   B. is recorded at 2 and 10 min.
   C. is a reliable indicator of future brain damage.
   D. records five different criteria.
   E. ranges from 5 to 25.

3. **Normal findings in a newborn baby include:**
   A. a mongolian blue spot.
   B. a strawberry naevus.
   C. vaginal blood loss.
   D. lanugo hair.
   E. erythema toxicum.

4. **In the transition from fetal circulation to neonatal circulation in a healthy baby:**
   A. the foramen ovale closes in the first 24 hours.
   B. the blood in the ductus arteriosus continues to flow from right to left until closure.
   C. the pulmonary artery resistance increases.
   D. the ductus arteriosus shuts in response to the increase in oxygen.
   E. blood continues to flow in the umbilical vessels for up to 48 hours.

1. **ABCDE**

   The embryonic phase of development occurs during first 12 weeks in utero. The fetal phase lasts from 12 weeks to delivery. The neonatal period is the first 28 days of life of a newborn infant of any gestation. The 1st year of life is infancy. The neonatal mortality rate is the number of deaths in the first 28 days per 1000 live births. The perinatal mortality rate is the number of stillbirths and early (up to 7 days) neonatal deaths per 1000 total births.

2. **D**

   The Apgar score is a standardised assessment of the condition of a newborn at 1 and 5 minutes after delivery. Early Apgar scores are not good predictors of outcome, although at 10 minutes an Apgar score of less than 5 correlates with a poor outcome. The Apgar score assesses heart rate, respiratory effort, reflex irritability, muscle tone and colour. Each criterion is scored from 0 to 2, giving a minimum score of 0 and a maximum score of 10.

3. **ACDE**

   A mongolian blue spot is a patchy accumulation of pigment commonly occurring over the buttocks and lower back. Vaginal blood loss in baby girls is due to maternal oestrogen withdrawal. Lanugo hair covers all babies, particularly the more premature. Erythema toxicum is a common blotchy red rash in newborn babies. The cause is unknown. A strawberry naevus, a vascular malformation, appears over the first few months of life and is rarely present in the early neonatal period.

4. **AD**

   After delivery, the change from fetal to adult circulation occurs over the first 24 hours. With the first cries, the lungs inflate and the pulmonary vascular resistance drops. Blood flows easily into the pulmonary vascular bed and is oxygenated. The ductus arteriosus shuts in response to higher oxygen concentration and a decrease in circulating prostaglandin. The foramen ovale functionally closes very soon after birth. As the pulmonary vascular resistance decreases and the systemic vascular resistance rises blood will transiently flow from left to right through the ductus until it closes.

5. **In the first 24 hours after delivery:**
   A. the kidneys produce urine for the first time only after separation of the placenta.
   B. the lungs produce surfactant only after the physiological stress of birth.
   C. fetal haemoglobin releases more oxygen to the tissues than adult haemoglobin under the same conditions.
   D. liver glycogen is the only available energy source for the first 24 hours.
   E. cell-mediated immunity is the main protection for the baby against infection.

6. **There is an increased risk of neonatal respiratory difficulty:**
   A. following prolonged rupture of the membranes.
   B. in the infant of a diabetic mother.
   C. after elective pre-labour caesarean section delivery.
   D. with meconium-stained liquor.
   E. with a family history of asthma.

7. **The Apgar score assesses:**
   A. the heart rate.
   B. the colour of the baby.
   C. the Moro reflex.
   D. the severity of birth asphyxia.
   E. the depth of respiratory depression from maternal analgesia.

8. **Regarding the head of a newborn infant:**
   A. a cephalohaematoma will resolve within the first 24 hours of life.
   B. caput is due to oedema of the presenting part of the head.
   C. a cephalohaematoma is due to bleeding into the skin.
   D. overlapping of the skull bones is a normal finding.
   E. a cephalohaematoma should be drained.

5. **None of these – all false**

   The kidneys produce urine from very early in gestation and over the last trimester of pregnancy 90% of the amniotic fluid is fetal urine. The lung type 2 pneumatocytes produce surfactant from around the 10th week of gestation. Surfactant production is accelerated after birth. Fetal haemoglobin takes up oxygen at low oxygen tension but releases oxygen to the peripheral tissues less readily than adult haemoglobin. Liver glycogen stores provide a readily available energy source; however, in the absence of liver glycogen babies can switch to fat metabolism. Early immunity is mainly from maternally acquired immuno-globulin. Cell-mediated immunity requires exposure to anti-gens to generate a response.

6. **ABCD**

   Respiratory distress can be caused by surfactant deficiency, infection, congenital abnormality or transient tachypnoea of the newborn, or aspiration of amniotic fluid, blood or meconium into the lungs. Prolonged rupture of the mem-branes increases the risk of infection. Infants of diabetic mothers may have decreased surfactant production. Caesarean section before the onset of labour is associated with an increased risk of transient tachypnoea due to delayed clearance of lung fluid. Meconium aspirated into the lungs may cause a pneumonitis. A family history of asthma is not relevant.

7. **AB**

   The Apgar score makes use of five criteria in order to guide resuscitation. The Apgar score is not a diagnostic or prognostic tool. These criteria are heart rate, colour, response to stimulus, respiratory effort and muscle tone. A baby should not be exposed to a painful stimulus unnecessarily. Maternal opiates may affect the baby and this may be reflected in a low Apgar score.

8. **BD**

   Cephalohaematomas are common and are usually due to bleeding under the parietal periosteum. Swelling is restricted by the limits of the sutures. The haematoma should not be drained as this raises the infection risk. It takes several weeks for the blood to be absorbed. Caput is due to oedema of the presenting part and resolves rapidly. Moulding (overlapping of the sutures) facilitates delivery.

9. **When describing the skull of a newborn baby:**
   A. the anterior fontanelle is triangular.
   B. the frontal and parietal bones border the anterior fontanelle.
   C. the coronal suture joins the anterior and posterior fontanelle.
   D. the posterior fontanelle is at the meeting point of the lambdoid and sagittal sutures.
   E. a third fontanelle is abnormal.

10. **A healthy newborn baby boy may:**
    A. have erythema of the umbilical skin which extends on to the abdomen.
    B. produce breast milk.
    C. have a single palmar crease.
    D. have an umbilical hernia.
    E. vomit blood if breast feeding.

11. **In the mouth of a newborn normal findings include:**
    A. teeth.
    B. Ebstein pearls.
    C. tongue tie.
    D. submucous cleft.
    E. bifid uvula.

12. **The reflexes present in a newborn baby include:**
    A. the Moro reflex.
    B. the grasp reflex.
    C. the rooting reflex.
    D. the asymmetric tonic neck reflex.
    E. the Babinski reflex.

9. **BD**

The diamond-shaped anterior fontanelle is bordered by the frontal and parietal bones. The sagittal suture connects the anterior and posterior fontanelle – the coronal suture runs from the lateral angles of the anterior fontanelle. The posterior fontanelle lies at the meeting point of the lambdoid and sagittal sutures. The 3rd fontanelle may lie between the anterior and posterior fontanelle and is a normal variant but occurs with increased frequency in babies with Down syndrome.

10. **BCDE**

An umbilical 'flare' indicates infection and should be treated with antibiotics. Neonates may produce breast milk due to stimulation by maternal hormones. A single palmar crease, although common in Down syndrome, is a normal variant. An umbilical hernia will resolve and does not require any intervention. The commonest reason why babies vomit blood is because they swallowed maternal blood, either at delivery or from cracked nipples.

11. **ABC**

A few babies have teeth at delivery, and these should be removed if loose to prevent inhalation. Ebstein pearls are tiny epidermal cysts which occur on the hard palate and which disappear spontaneously. A tongue tie – where the frenulum extends to the tip of the tongue – rarely causes symptoms and should be left alone. A submucous cleft is not normal and may require repair as it interferes with speech and swallowing. A bifid uvula may indicate other midline abnormalities.

12. **ABCD**

The Moro reflex is elicited by allowing the head to fall backwards relative to the trunk – the arms abduct and extend. The palmar grasp is elicited when an examining finger is placed in the baby's palm – initiating a reflex grasp. The rooting reflex aids the baby in latching on to the nipple. The tonic neck reflex is elicited by turning the baby's head to one side, and the baby adopts a posture similar to a fencer. The plantar reflex is elicited by stroking the outer aspect of the sole of the foot and is only present once babies have lost their grasp reflexes.

13. **In the first 24 hours of life it is normal:**
    A. to lose 15% of the birth weight.
    B. not to pass meconium.
    C. to be jaundiced.
    D. to have blood sugar of 1 mmol/L.
    E. to have pink urine stains in the nappy.

14. **The following neonatal skin findings require no treatment or investigation:**
    A. erythema toxicum.
    B. milia.
    C. generalised purpuric rash.
    D. Staphylococcal spots.
    E. melanocytic naevi.

15. **A fractured clavicle in a newborn infant:**
    A. occurs more frequently in infants of diabetic mothers.
    B. requires treatment with a sling.
    C. is associated with an Erb's palsy.
    D. causes an asymmetrical Moro reflex.
    E. is not painful.

16. **The problems associated with birth asphyxia include:**
    A. necrotising enterocolitis.
    B. syndrome of inappropriate ADH secretion.
    C. haematuria.
    D. metabolic alkalosis.
    E. hypotension.

**13.  E**

Breast-fed babies may lose up to 12% of their birth weight by the 5th day and usually regain it by 10 days. Babies should pass urine and meconium within the first 24 hours. Delayed passage of meconium may indicate Hirschsprung's disease, meconium ileus or bowel atresia. Jaundice in the first 24 hours is always pathological and suggests infection or haemolysis. A blood sugar level below 2.6 mmol/L is abnormal. Pink urine stains may occur on the napkin because of urate crystals and are normal.

**14.  AB**

Erythema toxicum occurs in about 50% of babies and is a macular blotchy rash with white or yellow centre. It fades spontaneously. Milia are tiny white spots over the nose and chin. They are due to blocked sebaceous glands. A generalised purpuric rash will require further investigation – causes include thrombocytopenia and intrauterine infections. Staphylococcal spots require antibiotic treatment. A melanocytic naevus has the risk of malignant change and may require removal.

**15.  ACD**

Infants of diabetic mothers have an increased risk of traumatic delivery because of their large size. If much force has been used to deliver the baby, there can be damage to the upper cervical nerve roots causing an Erb's palsy. Treatment is with immobilisation as it is painful and gentle physiotherapy. Sometimes it may be detected by an asymmetrical Moro.

**16.  ABCE**

Birth asphyxia may cause damage to many organs as a result of the hypoxia and poor perfusion. Bowel wall ischaemic damage may predispose to development of necrotising enterocolitis when feeds are started. SIADH is a common occurrence after such an insult and the baby may require fluid restriction. Damage to the renal tract will present as haematuria and damage to myocardial tissue may reduce cardiac function and cause loss of autonomic control. The baby will be acidotic because of excess lactic acid, although it may hyperventilate and produce a compensatory respiratory alkalosis.

**17.** **The following are likely to occur after severe birth asphyxia:**
   **A.** seizures within the first 6 hours.
   **B.** a cord pH less than 7.05.
   **C.** an absent suck reflex.
   **D.** acute tubular necrosis.
   **E.** marked hypotonia.

**18.** **The following predispose to a baby being small for gestational age:**
   **A.** placental insufficiency.
   **B.** twin pregnancy.
   **C.** congenital infection.
   **D.** maternal diabetes.
   **E.** alcohol consumption.

**19.** **The small for gestational age newborn baby is at an increased risk of:**
   **A.** hypoglycaemia.
   **B.** polycythaemia.
   **C.** hypothermia.
   **D.** hypothyroidism.
   **E.** cardiac abnormalities.

**20.** **There is an increased chance of a baby being large for gestational age if:**
   **A.** the mother is large and heavy.
   **B.** the mother is hypertensive.
   **C.** the baby has Down syndrome.
   **D.** the baby has an insulin-secreting tumour.
   **E.** the mother has diabetes.

17. **ABCDE**

    A severely asphyxiated baby will show multi-organ damage to a variable extent. Poor prognostic signs are failure to establish spontaneous respirations and need for assisted ventilation, seizure activity within the first 6 hours, an absent suck reflex and profound hypotonia. Acute tubular necrosis is certainly a sign of a major ischaemic event. There will often be good recovery of renal function.

18. **ABCDE**

    All these factors can result in an infant who is small for gestation. Multiple pregnancies produce smaller babies often because of a degree of placental insufficiency. Congenitally infected babies tend to be small for gestation. Maternal diabetes, although classically causing an infant to be large for gestation, will cause the opposite if there is poor placental function and a compromised fetus. The effect of alcohol on the fetus includes marked growth impairment, especially that of the brain.

19. **ABC**

    Babies who are small for gestational age may have had poor placental supply for some time. They have little fat and are therefore at risk of hypoglycaemia and hypothermia. If there has been poor placental oxygen transfer, they may have compensated with polycythaemia. They are not at risk of hypothyroidism or any more likely to have a cardiac lesion. Indeed some babies with cardiac lesions are large for dates.

20. **ADE**

    Down syndrome babies tend to be smaller. Hypertensive mothers can have poor placental function and the baby be small for gestation. If a mother is large, she tends to have large babies. As insulin is a growth hormone, babies with an insulin-secreting tumour (nesidioblastoma) can be very large. Infants of diabetic mothers who have been exposed to high levels of circulating glucose will switch on their own insulin production to maintain euglycaemia, thus exposing themselves to the growth stimulus of the insulin in utero.

**21.** **Hypoplastic lungs are typically found in babies who have:**
   **A.** diaphragmatic hernia.
   **B.** congenital muscular disorders.
   **C.** renal agenesis.
   **D.** been delivered following rupture of the membranes before 20 weeks' gestation.
   **E.** a congenital infection.

**22.** **The incidence of idiopathic respiratory distress syndrome is increased in:**
   **A.** premature infants.
   **B.** infants of mothers who were given steroids.
   **C.** premature boys compared to premature girls.
   **D.** asphyxiated term babies.
   **E.** prolonged rupture of the membranes.

**23.** **Idiopathic respiratory distress syndrome is characterised by:**
   **A.** reduced $PaCO_2$ due to hyperventilation.
   **B.** increasing oxygen requirement to maintain normal partial pressure oxygen in the blood.
   **C.** surfactant deficiency.
   **D.** patchy opacification on a CXR.
   **E.** initial deterioration over the first 48 hours.

**24.** **Respiratory distress syndrome is exacerbated by:**
   **A.** hypothermia.
   **B.** acidosis.
   **C.** hypoxia.
   **D.** meconium aspiration.
   **E.** withholding enteral feeds.

21. **ACD**

A space-occupying lesion within the thorax (e.g. a diaphrag-matic hernia) will prevent the lungs from growing and developing normally. In utero the normal fetal lung is partially inflated with lung fluid to allow fetal breathing which is necessary for normal lung development. In the absence of fluid *surrounding* the baby as in renal agenesis or premature rupture of the membranes the thorax of the baby is compressed and the resulting restriction of fetal breathing movements causes a failure of lung growth. Congenital muscular disorders can cause polyhydramnios as a result of absent swallowing, but the lungs are usually developed. Congenital infection does not cause lung hypoplasia.

22. **AC**

Idiopathic respiratory distress syndrome (IRDS) of prematurity results from a lack of surfactant. Surfactant production is increased by giving the mother steroids before delivery and is also increased if the baby is stressed – as in prolonged rupture of the membranes. Boys are more at risk of IRDS than girls of equivalent gestation. Asphyxiated term infants do not have problems with RDS, but severe acidosis does decrease surfactant production.

23. **BCE**

The clinical picture of untreated RDS is one of increasing respiratory effort with grunting, recession and tachypnoea. Rising levels of $CO_2$ or falling arterial oxygen levels may make ventilation necessary. The baby's oxygen requirement is a guide to the severity of the lung disease. The typical CXR of IRDS has a diffuse hazy or ground-glass appearance with a prominent air bronchogram pattern. In IRDS a baby's condition may deteriorate over the first 48 hours and then plateau before improvement occurs.

24. **ABCD**

The production of surfactant can be switched off by hypo-thermia, acidosis and hypoxia. Meconium aspiration can also interfere with surfactant production and some centres use surfactant in the critically ill baby who has meconium aspiration syndrome. Withholding enteral feeds reduces the risks to the baby of a full stomach compromising the diaphragmatic function and will reduce the risk of aspiration.

25. **Early clinical signs of respiratory distress syndrome are:**
    A. a respiratory rate greater than 60 breaths/min.
    B. expiratory grunting.
    C. central cyanosis if breathing air.
    D. intercostal recession.
    E. pyrexia.

26. **A newborn baby of 28 weeks' gestation with severe respiratory distress syndrome:**
    A. should be intubated and ventilated.
    B. requires surfactant therapy via a nasogastric tube.
    C. should have an arterial catheter inserted.
    D. has a less than 50% chance of survival.
    E. will not require any analgesia.

27. **Transient tachypnoea of the newborn:**
    A. occurs in 15% of full-term babies.
    B. can be diagnosed if onset occurs up to 48 hours post delivery.
    C. is caused by delayed absorption of fetal lung fluid.
    D. occurs more commonly in babies delivered by caesarean section.
    E. cannot be clearly differentiated from early pneumonia.

28. **Organisms implicated in transplacentally acquired pneumonia include:**
    A. cytomegalovirus.
    B. listeria.
    C. Pneumococci.
    D. varicella.
    E. rubella.

**25. ABCD**

The early signs are of the increased respiratory effort. In an attempt to reduce collapse of the alveoli during expiration, the baby tries to maintain partial inflation of the lungs and so expires against a partially closed glottis. This causes a grunting noise. As a result of generating a significant negative intrathoracic pressure, the softer structures recess. Untreated the babies would become cyanosed. IRDS does not cause a pyrexia.

**26. AC**

Many units would electively intubate babies of less than 30 weeks' gestation with any signs of respiratory difficulty because of the high risk of respiratory problems and the poor reserve these babies have. Surfactant therapy must be given directly into the lungs via an endotracheal tube. Such babies need to be closely monitored ideally with an (umbilical) arterial catheter. Babies have a good chance of survival at 28 weeks – approximately 80%; however, as they are subjected to many stressful procedures during their initial problems, they should receive analgesia.

**27. CDE**

Transient tachypnoea of the newborn (TTN) occurs because of delayed clearance of lung fluid. TTN occurs in less than 5% of babies, depending on the elective caesarean section rate. After elective caesarean section, TTN may develop as babies have not been subjected to the normal mechanisms that help to clear lung fluid during delivery. TTN becomes clinically apparent shortly after birth and has usually resolved with 24 hours. CXR may show streaky change and fluid in the horizontal fissure. It may be difficult to differentiate between the causes of neonatal respiratory distress.

**28. ABDE**

The congenitally acquired viral infections can cause pneumonia – cytomegalovirus (CMV), varicella and rubella have all been implicated. The commonest of these is CMV pneumonitis. Listeria can also cause a pneumonia and must always be considered in the premature baby with meconium-stained liquor. Pneumococci cause pneumonia but this is acquired by the transvaginal route.

**29. A newborn infant is at increased risk of pneumonia if:**
   A. there was prolonged rupture of the membranes.
   B. the maternal vaginal tract is colonised with Group B Streptococci.
   C. he inhales amniotic fluid at the time of delivery.
   D. he has a tracheo-oesophageal fistula.
   E. he is a carrier for the cystic fibrosis gene.

**30. Factors associated with bronchopulmonary dysplasia include:**
   A. a positive family history.
   B. prematurity.
   C. mechanical ventilation.
   D. history of respiratory distress syndrome.
   E. pulmonary infection.

**31. A baby born at 31 weeks' gestation has recurrent apnoeic episodes. This may:**
   A. be normal.
   B. indicate infection.
   C. be treated with caffeine.
   D. be due to too high oxygen concentration.
   E. require ventilation.

**32. An indication of fetal distress in labour is:**
   A. a scalp pH of 7.35.
   B. fresh meconium staining of the liquor.
   C. a fetal heart rate of 200 beats/min.
   D. maternal pyrexia.
   E. significant beat-to-beat variability of heart rate.

**29.  ABCD**

Prolonged rupture of membranes (greater than 24 hours) increases the chance of transvaginal infection as the physical barrier has been breached. If the maternal tract is colonised with any pathological bacteria (e.g. Group B haemolytic Streptococci), this increases the risk of transmission of infection to the baby. If the baby gasps during delivery and inhales amniotic fluid, an aspiration pneumonia may result even if the amniotic fluid is not infected. A tracheo-oesophageal fistula will allow gastrointestinal contents to enter the lungs more easily. Carriers for the CF gene are not at an increased risk.

**30.  BCDE**

They are easily damaged by the barotrauma of mechanical ventilation necessary in severe RDS. Many other factors contribute: high oxygen tension is thought to damage the lungs, as does infection. The definition of bronchopulmonary dysplasia is variable, but is commonly taken as a persisting oxygen requirement at 36 weeks' corrected gestation.

**31.  ABCE**

Apnoea of prematurity is well recognised but should only be diagnosed after excluding more serious causes. In neonates recurrent apnoea is a common reason for performing an infection screen. Some babies may require ventilation. Caffeine is a respiratory stimulant and is used with good effect.

**32.  BC**

Mothers are monitored during labour in an attempt to detect any fetal compromise. The fetal heart rate is monitored either intermittently with a pinnard or continuously with a trans-abdominal transducer, or an electrode attached to the scalp. Tachycardia and decreased beat-to-beat variability are possible signs of fetal distress. A fetal scalp blood sample pH $< 7.25$ suggests fetal distress. If a baby is distressed, it may defecate in utero causing the liquor to be stained with meconium. Maternal pyrexia usually indicates maternal infection, but is not evidence of fetal distress.

**33.** **Meconium aspiration syndrome:**
   A. occurs more commonly in asphyxiated infants than an uncomplicated delivery.
   B. increases the risk of a pneumothorax.
   C. presents as a ground-glass appearance on CXR.
   D. is caused by plugging of the airways by meconium.
   E. resolves over 24–48 hours.

**34.** **A neonate who is intubated and ventilated is at increased risk of developing:**
   A. inguinal herniae.
   B. a pneumothorax.
   C. an intraventricular haemorrhage.
   D. pneumonia.
   E. bronchopulmonary dysplasia.

**35.** **A preterm baby of 30 weeks' gestation is intubated and ventilated. On the 2nd day of life he suddenly deteriorates. The differential diagnosis includes:**
   A. an intraventricular haemorrhage.
   B. a blocked endotracheal tube.
   C. a pulmonary haemorrhage.
   D. pneumonia.
   E. self-extubation.

**36.** **Clinical features of heart failure in the newborn include:**
   A. tachypnoea.
   B. warm peripheries.
   C. hepatomegaly.
   D. sweating.
   E. swollen ankles.

33. **ABD**

Meconium aspiration syndrome occurs when a baby inhales meconium-stained liquor into the lungs. Meconium is viscid and causes a chemical pneumonitis with plugging of the airways. A pneumothorax may occur if there is air trapping and over-distension of a part of the lung. The CXR shows patchy opacification with areas of collapse and hyperinflation. The clinical picture resolves over many days.

34. **ABCDE**

High intrathoracic pressure during assisted ventilation can result in pulmonary air leaks. Sudden changes in intrathoracic pressure are transmitted to the great vessels and the risk of intraventricular bleeds is increased. Prematurity is associated with an increased risk of inguinal hernia. An endotracheal tube increases the risk of bacterial colonisation of the lungs. Long-term infection and barotrauma may lead to lung damage and development of bronchopulmonary dysplasia.

35. **ABCE**

The important causes of sudden deterioration are mechanical such as a blocked or dislodged tube, a problem with the ventilator circuit or with the baby. A tension pneumothorax will cause mediastinal shift, in addition to respiratory compromise. A pulmonary haemorrhage will cause problems with gas transfer and possibly hypovolaemia. An intraventricular bleed can cause sudden deterioration due to blood loss. A pneumonia tends to cause a gradual change in condition.

36. **ACD**

Heart failure causes increased rate and effort of breathing as the lungs are less compliant because of excess interstitial fluid. The peripheral perfusion is decreased and there will be peripheral vasoconstriction in an attempt to maintain perfusion of vital tissues. The peripheries are cold and clammy, with sluggish capillary return. Feeding is difficult due to breath-lessness. Feeding also requires energy which puts further demands on the myocardial function. There may be evidence of venous overload with hepatomegaly. Neonates do not develop ankle oedema.

37. **At the discharge check from the maternity hospital a well baby is found to have a heart murmur. The appropriate management is:**
    A. to postpone discharge for 48 hours and observe the baby.
    B. to measure his blood pressure in all four limbs.
    C. to record an electrocardiogram.
    D. to request an urgent echocardiogram.
    E. to request a CXR.

38. **A well baby is centrally cyanosed at 24 hours old. The differential diagnosis includes:**
    A. transposition of the great arteries.
    B. Fallot's tetralogy.
    C. aortic stenosis.
    D. a ventricular septal defect.
    E. pulmonary atresia.

39. **A baby presents in heart failure at 5 days of age. The baby is not centrally cyanosed. The differential diagnosis includes:**
    A. atrial septal defect.
    B. Fallot's tetralogy.
    C. hypoplastic left heart.
    D. coarctation of the aorta.
    E. tricuspid atresia.

40. **A well baby has difficulty sucking. Causes for this could be:**
    A. micrognathia.
    B. dystrophia myotonica.
    C. cleft palate.
    D. Prader–Willi syndrome.
    E. bulbar palsy.

**37.  BCE**

It is quite common to hear murmurs in neonates, which may be pathological or innocent. The difficulty is in deciding whether to investigate further in an otherwise well baby with no signs of cardiac disease. The majority of murmurs will be innocent and babies with abnormal cardiac anatomy may well have no murmur in the immediate postnatal period. Most important abnormalities can be detected with a CXR, by measuring the blood pressure in all four limbs and by taking an ECG.

**38.  AE**

Central cyanosis is detected when there is more than 5 g/dl of reduced haemoglobin in the circulation. In a well baby a respiratory cause is unlikely. Cardiac causes of cyanosis must have a right to left shunt, with deoxygenated blood passing into the systemic circulation. In pulmonary atresia the blood passes through a persistent atrial opening. In transposition of the great arteries there is persistent circulation of deoxygenated blood around the systemic circulation. In aortic stenosis and large ventricular septal defects there is no right to left shunt in neonates. In tetralogy of Fallot the neonate is usually not cyanosed – cyanosis, due to progressive right ventricular outflow obstruction, develops later during the 1st year of life.

**39.  CDE**

Cardiac failure results from cardiac lesions, which result in low- or high-output states. In low-output failure there may be obstruction to outflow as in a coarctation or critical aortic stenosis, inadequate muscle pump as in hypoplastic heart or lack of blood flow to the heart as in right-sided lesions, such as tricuspid atresia. In the latter case, the child would also be cyanosed. An atrial septal defect alone rarely causes heart failure.

**40.  ABCDE**

Anatomical disorders that cause difficulty with feeding include a small chin (micrognathia), cleft palate or large tongue. Lack of power occurs in dystrophia myotonica and is part of the problem in Prader–Willi syndrome, as well as central motor control. A bulbar palsy is rare in neonates, but can occur after severe birth asphyxia.

41. **Necrotising enterocolitis presents with:**
    A. a distended abdomen.
    B. blood-stained faeces.
    C. septicaemia.
    D. bilious vomits.
    E. perforation of small bowel.

42. **The risk of developing necrotising enterocolitis is increased in:**
    A. breast-fed babies.
    B. asphyxiated babies.
    C. premature babies.
    D. infants who have the umbilical artery catheterised.
    E. infants who have had no milk feeds.

43. **The causes for failure to pass meconium in the first 24 hours of life include:**
    A. cystic fibrosis.
    B. hyperthyroidism.
    C. Hirschsprung's disease.
    D. hiatus hernia.
    E. galactosaemia.

44. **A baby is jaundiced at 12 hours old. The causes to consider are:**
    A. sepsis.
    B. haemolytic disease of the newborn.
    C. biliary atresia.
    D. congenital spherocytosis.
    E. hypothyroidism.

**41. ABCDE**

Necrotising enterocolitis (NEC) is usually a disease of the premature neonate. The aetiology is unknown. The abdomen becomes distended – there is an ileus. There may be large bilious vomits. There may be blood loss from the inflamed mucosa. Secondary infection follows the invasion of the bowel wall by gas-forming organisms. The baby may become septicaemic and bowel perforation may occur at points of marked inflammation.

**42. BCD**

The use of breast milk is protective, although it does not prevent NEC. A baby who has not been orally fed will not usually develop NEC. There is risk of ischaemic damage to the bowel mucosa following severe birth asphyxia. An umbilical artery catheter may affect the blood supply to the gut from the superior mesenteric axis and may also cause microemboli, resulting in bowel ischaemia. Premature babies are prone to episodes of hypotension and infection which increase the risk of NEC.

**43. AC**

The timing of the first dirty nappy is always noted by the midwifery staff. 95% of normal infants will pass meconium in the first 24 hours. Delay in passage may be due to viscid meconium, or a meconium plug as in cystic fibrosis. In Hirschsprung's disease there is a failure of neuronal migration causing aganglionosis of the rectum, which extends proximally for a variable distance. Proximal to the abnormal segment the gut can become grossly distended. *Hypo*thyroidism can present with neonatal constipation. Hiatus hernia and galactosaemia do not cause delayed passage of meconium.

**44. ABD**

Jaundice within the first 24 hours of life is always pathological and needs urgent assessment. If the jaundice is secondary to excess haemolysis, urgent treatment may be required to prevent hyperbilirubinaemia. Haemolysis may result from maternal antibodies to fetal red cells as in rhesus or ABO incompatibility (haemolytic disease of the newborn) or destruction of abnormal cells as in congenital spherocytosis. Severe sepsis may also cause profound haemolysis. Biliary atresia and hypothyroidism will not cause problems in the first 24 hours.

**45.** **The investigations that should be done to elucidate the cause of jaundice in a 24-hour-old baby include:**
   **A.** the Guthrie test.
   **B.** serum conjugated bilirubin level.
   **C.** full blood count.
   **D.** indirect Coombs test.
   **E.** urine analysis for reducing substances.

**46.** **A 15-day-old baby has a conjugated hyperbilirubinaemia. The differential diagnosis includes:**
   **A.** breast milk jaundice.
   **B.** hyperthyroidism.
   **C.** ABO incompatibility.
   **D.** congenital cytomegalovirus infection.
   **E.** Crigler–Najjar syndrome.

**47.** **The clinical features that would suggest an obstructive cause in a jaundiced baby are:**
   **A.** absent bilirubin in the urine.
   **B.** lack of pigment in the stools.
   **C.** increased gamma glutamyl transferase level.
   **D.** evidence of a bleeding tendency.
   **E.** family history of alpha-1-antitrypsin deficiency.

**48.** **Polycythaemia in the neonatal period is associated with the following:**
   **A.** Down syndrome.
   **B.** the donor twin in a twin-to-twin transfusion.
   **C.** maternal diabetes.
   **D.** intrauterine growth retardation.
   **E.** respiratory distress syndrome.

**45. C**

A full blood count may reveal a low haemoglobin. Thrombocytopenia or neutropenia may suggest infection. Reducing substances may be found in the urine in galactosaemia – infants may deteriorate rapidly with sepsis, jaundice, vomiting and diarrhoea, but usually not until the end of the 1st week of life. The Guthrie test is done on days 5 or 6. Conjugated hyperbilirubinaemia does not present in the first few days of life. The *direct* Coombs test detects the presence of antibodies to red cell surface markers.

**46. D**

Breast milk or physiological jaundice and ABO incompatibility cause an unconjugated hyperbilirubinaemia. Hypothyroidism causes both a conjugated and unconjugated hyperbilirubinaemia, but hyperthyroidism does not. Crigler–Najjar is caused by an absence of glucuronyl transferase and the jaundice is unconjugated and severe. Congenital viral infections, particularly cytomegalovirus infection, cause a hepatitis with a conjugated hyperbilirubinaemia and abnormal liver function tests.

**47. BCDE**

Conjugated hyperbilirubinaemia is caused either by intra- or extrahepatic cholestasis. Extrahepatic cholestasis can cause a complete obstruction to passage of bile. Intrahepatic cholestasis tends not to be complete and presents with a hepatitis picture with elevated GGT and alanine aminotransferase levels, such as in alpha-1-antitrypsin deficiency. Obstructive jaundice presents with pale stools and dark urine. There is no bilirubin in the stools, which are pale. There is excretion of bilirubin in the urine. Vitamin K malabsorption may lead to a coagulopathy.

**48. ACDE**

Polycythaemia is a cause of neonatal morbidity. A high haematocrit increases the viscosity of blood and the resulting poor capillary perfusion may cause respiratory distress, cerebral ischaemia and gut ischaemia. Down syndrome is a well-known association. Intrauterine hypoxia will increase red cell production as in intrauterine growth retardation and in some infants of diabetic mothers. The recipient twin in a twin-to-twin transfusion is the one at risk of polycythaemia.

49. **The following tests are used to detect the accompanying diagnosis:**
    A. Kleihauer and feto-maternal transfusion.
    B. hyperoxia test and respiratory distress syndrome.
    C. test feed and hiatus hernia.
    D. Apt's test and renal tubular acidosis.
    E. 'double bubble' on plain abdominal film and jejunal atresia.

50. **Haemorrhagic disease of the newborn:**
    A. is secondary to a low prothrombin.
    B. can present up to 6 months of life.
    C. is treated with protamine sulphate.
    D. is prevented by administering vitamin E to all newborn babies.
    E. can result in intracerebral haemorrhage.

51. **Regarding rhesus disease:**
    A. it is prevented by injecting all babies of rhesus-negative mothers with anti-D immunoglobulin.
    B. the severity of the disease increases with each affected pregnancy.
    C. fetal anaemia is caused by intravascular destruction of red cells.
    D. hydrops fetalis is caused by kidney failure.
    E. the fetal anaemia may be treated with injection of red cells into the fetal abdomen.

52. **A newborn baby has profound thrombocytopenia. The causes include:**
    A. cytomegalovirus infection.
    B. autoimmune neonatal thrombocytopenia.
    C. maternal ingestion of warfarin.
    D. alloimmune neonatal thrombocytopenia.
    E. gram-negative septicaemia.

**49. A**

Fetal cells are able to resist acid elution and denaturation by sodium hydroxide, which forms the basis for the Kleihauer test, which is used to detect evidence of feto-maternal haemorrhage. Apt's test is used after neonatal haematemesis to distinguish gastrointestinal haemorrhage and swallowed maternal blood. A test feed is to diagnose pyloric stenosis. The hyperoxia test is used to aid diagnosis in congenital heart disease. A plain abdominal X-ray film which shows a 'double bubble' is diagnostic of duodenal atresia.

**50. BE**

Haemorrhagic disease of the newborn (HDN) is caused by vitamin K deficiency. It classically presents in the first few days of life but can occur up to 6 months postnatal age. HDN can present with haemorrhage in any system, particularly the gastrointestinal tract, lungs or brain. Treatment is to administer vitamin K and infuse fresh blood plasma.

**51. BE**

Any transfer of fetal blood from a rhesus-positive baby (either at or prior to delivery) to a rhesus-negative mother will result in the production of antibodies, which may then cross the placenta and cause destruction of fetal red cells in the spleen. The process becomes worse with each affected pregnancy. An affected fetus can become anaemic, develop heart failure (hydrops fetalis) and die. Rhesus disease is prevented by injecting all rhesus-negative *mothers* after miscarriages and after the delivery of a rhesus-positive baby with anti-D immuno-globulin. Intrauterine transfusions may be given via the cord vessels or by intra-abdominal injection.

**52. ABDE**

Congenital viral infections – particularly cytomegalovirus – cause thrombocytopenia. Acute gram-negative sepsis can present with a consumptive coagulopathy. Alloimmune thrombocytopenia results from the transplacental passage of antibodies from a platelet antigen-negative mother to her platelet antigen-positive (98% of the population) fetus. The most common cause of autoimmune thrombocytopenia, caused by the passive transfer of maternal antibodies, is maternal idiopathic thrombocytopenia purpura.

53. **A severely hydropic infant is about to be delivered. Complications to be prepared for are:**
    A. pulmonary hypoplasia.
    B. abdominal ascites.
    C. polycythaemia.
    D. heart failure.
    E. laryngeal oedema.

54. **Hydrops fetalis is associated with:**
    A. beta-thalassaemia.
    B. diaphragmatic hernia.
    C. paroxysmal supraventricular tachycardia.
    D. OA materno-fetal blood group incompatibility.
    E. Turner syndrome.

55. **Periventricular haemorrhage (PVH) in neonates occurs:**
    A. with increasing frequency in the post-gestational babies.
    B. classically occurs in utero.
    C. has an increased incidence in ventilated babies.
    D. occurs within the cerebral cortex.
    E. causes neurological problems in all affected babies.

56. **Bacterial meningitis in the neonate:**
    A. is less common than in the general paediatric population.
    B. is caused by organisms similar to those in older children with meningitis.
    C. causes neurological impairment in 70–80% of survivors.
    D. is diagnosed when the CSF protein level is over 500 mg/L.
    E. causes ratio of CSF:blood glucose to be greater than 0.75.

**53. ABDE**
A severely hydropic infant will be grossly oedematous. The first priority is to obtain adequate ventilation and perfusion. Pleural effusions may be long-standing and result in pulmonary hypoplasia. It may be necessary to insert bilateral chest drains. Abdominal ascites may also require to be drained. There may be significant upper airway oedema and intubation can be difficult due to laryngeal oedema. Severe anaemia may require emergency transfusion.

**54. BCE**
Severe anaemia, heart failure, hypoproteinaemia and venous obstruction are all recognised causes of hydrops. In a significant number of cases, no cause is found. Supraventricular tachycardia may result in heart failure and hydrops. A diaphragmatic hernia may cause cardiac compromise and hydrops. There is a known association with many chromosomal defects. Severe anaemia does not occur in OA blood group incompatibility in utero. Severe anaemia in beta-thalassaemia occurs only in the postnatal period. Homozygous alpha-thalassaemia may present with hydrops fetalis.

**55. C**
Periventricular haemorrhage occurs in premature babies; and haemorrhage occurs in the germinal matrix in the floor of the lateral ventricles. They rarely occur in utero, but usually within the 1st week of life. Rapid changes in blood pressure will increase the risk of an intraventricular bleed. Thus a sick, ventilated premature baby is at high risk. A small bleed may cause no long-term problems. A large bleed may extend into the brain tissue and cause subsequent neurological handicap.

**56. None of these – all false**
Bacterial meningitis in the neonate is commoner than in the general population and may present insidiously. The infecting organisms include Group B Streptococci, *E. coli* and listeria. A sick neonate should have a lumbar puncture unless too unwell to tolerate the procedure. CSF protein levels up to 1200 mg/L are normal in the neonate. The CSF:blood glucose ratio is greater than 0.75 in the normal neonate. The CSF glucose will be lower in bacterial meningitis. Long-term sequelae of meningitis occur only in 30–40% – the commonest is deafness.

**57. Causes of neonatal convulsions are:**
 A. asphyxia.
 B. hypoglycaemia.
 C. hypomagnesaemia.
 D. maternal drug addiction.
 E. hyperkalaemia.

**58. You are called to see a two-day-old jittery baby. The causes to consider are:**
 A. maternal diabetes.
 B. fetal alcohol syndrome.
 C. maternal hyperparathyroidism.
 D. maternal thyrotoxicosis.
 E. congenital adrenal hyperplasia.

**59. Neural tube defects:**
 A. occur with a frequency of 2 per 10 000 births.
 B. have a genetic predisposition.
 C. result from abnormal development of the neural tube at 3–4 months' gestation.
 D. can be detected antenatally by low-serum alpha-fetoprotein levels.
 E. are treated with folic acid.

**60. Rickets of prematurity:**
 A. is associated with chronic respiratory distress.
 B. is prevented by administration of vitamin D.
 C. is less severe in infants fed with breast milk compared to formula-fed infants.
 D. can result in spontaneous fractures.
 E. is caused by a substrate deficiency.

**57. ABCD**

Convulsions in the neonatal period may result from a variety of biochemical abnormalities such as hypoglycaemia, hypocalcaemia and hypomagnesaemia. Acute drug withdrawal can cause convulsions and affected babies may need more gradual drug withdrawal. The severe neonatal asphyxia will commonly cause seizures.

**58. ABCD**

Jitteriness can be an exaggerated startle response or may have an underlying pathological cause. Hypoglycaemia occurs in infants of diabetic mothers. Drug withdrawal as in infants of alcoholics causes tremor. Maternal hyperparathyroidism may suppress fetal parathyroid production and cause fetal hypocalcaemia and tremor. In thyrotoxicosis maternal thyroid-stimulating antibodies can cross the placenta and cause transient neonatal hyperthyroidism. Infants with congenital adrenal hyperplasia may develop hyponatraemia and hypoglycaemia but not usually on the second day of life.

**59. B**

The incidence of neural tube defects is 2 per 1000 births with wide regional variation. There is a genetic predisposition and the risk is increased for subsequent pregnancies after one affected child. The aetiology is multifactorial but the incidence is decreased by ingestion of folic acid prior to conception and during the first few weeks of development. The neural tube is formed between 3 and 4 weeks' gestation. The screening programme picks up cases by detecting an *elevated* serum alphafetoprotein level and offering detailed scanning to these mothers. Once the defect has occurred, it cannot be treated. The decision on whether to terminate the pregnancy will depend on the severity of the lesion.

**60. ADE**

Rickets, or metabolic bone disease of prematurity, results from decreased bone mineralisation. If the ribs are affected by softening, there may be further respiratory compromise and a risk of spontaneous fractures. Rickets cannot be prevented solely by administering vitamin D, but it is important to include this with calcium and phosphate supplements. Breast milk contains less calcium and phosphate and so may require supplementation with formula milk.

# Minitest 2

1. **In Fallot's tetralogy:**
   A. cyanosis is present from birth.
   B. heart failure occurs during the first 6 weeks of life.
   C. there is a typical pansystolic murmur from the ventricular septal defect.
   D. a subclavian artery to pulmonary artery shunt will abolish cyanotic spells.
   E. correction of the defect is only possible by heart transplantation.

2. **The following skin conditions should be left to resolve without treatment:**
   A. neonatal erythema toxicum.
   B. impetigo.
   C. facial naevus flammaeus – 'stork mark'.
   D. seborrhoeic dermatitis.
   E. strawberry haemangioma.

3. **The following drugs may be given down an endotracheal tube during emergency resuscitation:**
   A. atropine.
   B. adrenaline.
   C. plasma.
   D. 8.4% sodium bicarbonate.
   E. 50% dextrose.

4. **The following findings are more likely to be due to child abuse than to have an innocent cause:**
   A. an unexplained long bone fracture in a toddler whose father is deaf and has a history of multiple long bone fractures in childhood.
   B. fractures of different ages affecting non-identical twins, aged 6 months.
   C. retinal haemorrhages after a fall from a bed on to the carpeted floor.
   D. three clearly defined, circular blisters, 1 cm in diameter, with a raised, reddened edge to the lesions, affecting the back of both hands and one buttock.
   E. perianal warts affecting a 6-month-old baby.

1. **D**

   In Fallot's tetralogy cyanosis is uncommon at birth unless there is severe pulmonary stenosis (PS). Cyanosis results from progressive muscularisation and obstruction of the right ventricular outflow tract. PS is protective against heart failure by preventing significant left to right shunting. The murmur is from the PS and not a pansystolic ventricular septal defect murmur. A Blalock–Taussig shunt provides constant pulmonary blood flow, abolishes cyanotic spells and encourages pulmonary artery growth. Total surgical correction is usually carried out during infancy.

2. **ACE**

   Erythema toxicum (neonatorum) is a blotchy, erythematous rash which comes and goes over the first 7–10 days of life. The 'stork mark' capillary naevus is seen over the eyelids, the nape of the neck and sometimes the bridge of the nose – the facial components usually disappear completely. Strawberry haemangioma usually resolve by 2 years. Seborrhoeic dermatitis causes cradle cap and may spread and become infected. Staphylococcal impetigo spreads rapidly and requires antibiotic treatment.

3. **AB**

   Atropine, adrenaline and naloxone may be given into the endotracheal tube in an emergency resuscitation before intravenous access has been obtained. Large volumes of plasma will flood the lungs. Sodium bicarbonate 8.4% and dextrose 50% are hypertonic and intensely irritant. All drugs and resuscitation fluids may be given by an intraosseous needle.

4. **BCD**

   Osteogenesis imperfecta is suggested by a family history of repeated fractures, blue sclerae, early-onset deafness or dentinogenesis imperfecta. Retinal haemorrhages and multiple fractures of different ages in relatively immobile infants are almost always caused by abuse. Minor falls on to carpeted floors rarely produce any injury. Cigarette burns produce typical lesions, as described in question D. Perianal warts may occur as a result of transmission of the virus at birth, during normal child care procedures or – and no one knows how frequently – from child sex abuse.

5. **An 8-year-old child is receiving inhaled budesonide in a dose of 200 μg twice daily for asthma. On this dose his asthma is under good control. He is at increased risk of:**
   A. adrenal insufficiency in times of acute illness.
   B. delayed puberty.
   C. reduced final height.
   D. osteoporosis.
   E. diabetes mellitus.

6. **When breast feeding:**
   A. feeding should be limited to no more than 15 min on each breast.
   B. a baby should be fed from both breasts at each feed.
   C. supplements of sterile water should be used postnatally to reduce the degree of jaundice.
   D. babies should be weaned on to formula milk at 4 months of age.
   E. iron and vitamin supplements should be given from 4 months of age.

7. **The following conditions are reliably diagnosed by mucosal biopsy:**
   A. sucrase deficiency.
   B. cystic fibrosis.
   C. giardiasis.
   D. *Helicobacter pylori* infection.
   E. Hirschsprung's disease.

8. **The following are diagnostic of Down syndrome:**
   A. Brushfield spots.
   B. single palmar crease.
   C. duodenal atresia.
   D. 47, XY + 21 karyotype.
   E. 46, XY + t (14q21q) karyotype.

5. **B**

Appropriate therapeutic doses of current inhaled steroids never induce adrenal insufficiency or diabetes. Systemically absorbed inhaled steroids are rapidly inactivated by first-pass hepatic metabolism. Final height in mild to moderate asthmatics is normal, though even in simple atopy puberty may be delayed. There is no evidence yet to show that inhaled steroids affect bone mineralisation in children.

6. **None of these – all false**

No artificial time limits should be imposed on the breast feeding baby. The hind milk is richer in fat and therefore higher in calories. Many babies will feed from only one breast at a feed. Supplementary water does not reduce neonatal jaundice and may reduce the baby's suckling, thus inhibiting lactation. Mothers should be encouraged to continue breast feeding for as much of the first year as possible. It is recommended that solids should not routinely be given before 4 months of age. For full-term healthy babies whose mothers are taking a good diet there is no requirement for supplementary iron or vitamins.

7. **ACDE**

Small intestinal disaccharidase enzyme activity may be measured on a jejunal biopsy specimen. Breath hydrogen estimation may also be useful after sugar loading. *Giardia lamblia*, a flagellated protozoa, may be seen on microscopy of jejunal fluid or biopsy. Giardia cysts may be found on stool microscopy. *H. pylori* may be seen on microscopy of a gastric mucosal biopsy. A urease test will confirm the diagnosis. In Hirschsprung's disease an excess of acetylcholine-producing nerve endings will be seen on staining a mucosal biopsy. Absence of ganglion cells will be seen on deeper biopsy. Cystic fibrosis is not diagnosed by mucosal biopsy.

8. **DE**

The individual physical abnormalities of Down syndrone of themselves are not diagnostic of the condition. The combination of physical characteristics and the neurological abnormality (hypotonia) together make a clinical diagnosis of Down syndrome relatively simple. A Down syndrome karyotype, either classical or involving a translocation, is diagnostic of the condition.

9. **Most (more than 75%) of children of 4 years will be able to:**
    A. remain continent of urine by day.
    B. stand steadily on one foot.
    C. copy a circle.
    D. identify correctly three out of four primary colours.
    E. use prepositions.

10. **In congenital spherocytosis:**
    A. there is an increased risk of hyperbilirubinaemia in the neonatal period.
    B. there is an X-linked recessive mode of inheritance.
    C. there will be splenomegaly.
    D. red cell osmotic fragility will be decreased.
    E. there is an increased risk of developing gallstones.

11. **Increased susceptibility to bacterial infection is associated with:**
    A. sickle cell disease.
    B. hypogammaglobulinaemia.
    C. splenectomy.
    D. neutrophil count below $1 \times 10^9/L$.
    E. chronic granulomatous disease.

12. **Metabolic causes of vomiting include:**
    A. hyponatraemia.
    B. hypoglycaemia.
    C. ketoacidosis.
    D. hyperammoniaemia.
    E. hypercalcaemia.

9. **ACDE**

A child of 4 years will be dry by day – usually necessary before starting at nursery. Copying a circle is achieved by 3 years, a cross by 4 years and a square by $4\frac{1}{2}$ years. Standing or hopping on one leg for more than 10 s is achieved by 5–6 years. By 3 years 50% of children will be able to identify three out of four primary colours correctly. Prepositions are used by 3 years.

10. **ACE**

Spherocytes are common in the peripheral blood film of neonates. Diagnosis in this age group may therefore be difficult unless there is a positive family history. Inheritance is autosomal dominant. Spherocytosis results in increased red cell breakdown adding to the load of bilirubin to be conjugated and excreted. Formal diagnosis is by demonstrating an increased red cell osmotic fragility. In haemolytic conditions there is an increased risk of pigment gallstones formation.

11. **ABCDE – all of these**

In sickle cell disease there is a risk of septicaemia and pneumonia (Haemophilus and Pneumococcus) and osteomyelitis (*Staph. aureus* and Salmonella). After splenectomy, there is susceptibility to infection with encapsulated organisms – Pneumococcus and Haemophilus. Immunisation prior to surgery and lifelong prophylactic oral penicillin V is usually advised. Children with low levels of immunoglobulins have increased susceptibility, particularly to bacterial infection. Absolute neutropenia – a count of less than $1 \times 10^9/L$ – indicates a risk of spontaneous sepsis, particularly with gram-negative organisms. In chronic granulomatous disease (CGD) there is defective killing of organisms by neutrophils and skin, lung, lymph node and chronic GI infections are common.

12. **ACDE**

Hyponatraemia ($Na^+ < 120\,mmol/L$) is associated with intracellular fluid shift and cerebral oedema, characterised by recurrent vomiting and altered consciousness level. Diabetic ketoacidosis is associated with vomiting and severe abdominal pain, which resolves once the ketoacidosis is treated with fluids and insulin. Hyperammoniaemia is characterised by profuse vomiting and a metabolic alkalosis. Significant hypercalcaemia is associated with severe vomiting.

**13. Radiant heat loss from a newborn preterm infant can be minimised by:**
 A. drying the baby carefully.
 B. placing the baby in an incubator.
 C. increasing the humidity within the incubator.
 D. increasing the air temperature within the incubator.
 E. placing an overhead heater over the incubator.

**14. In classical, type 1, distal renal tubular acidosis there is:**
 A. failure to thrive.
 B. nephrocalcinosis.
 C. hypochloraemia.
 D. respiratory depression.
 E. a normal anion gap.

**15. The following are true with regard to blood pressure in childhood:**
 A. when taking measurements, the inflatable portion of the cuff should cover not more than 50% of the length of the humerus.
 B. at any given age there is no significant difference in the blood pressure between sexes in prepubertal children.
 C. in a hypertensive child the blood pressure may be significantly higher in the left arm than the right arm.
 D. hypertension in children is due to renal pathology in over 75% of cases.
 E. a systolic blood pressure of 120 mmHg in an asymptomatic 1-year-old child requires immediate treatment.

**16. Tumour lysis syndrome:**
 A. is characterised by hyperkalaemia.
 B. is characterised by hyperuricaemia.
 C. is characterised by hyperphosphataemia.
 D. is reduced in severity by treatment with allopurinol.
 E. is reduced in severity by moderate fluid restriction.

13. **BE**

Radiant heat loss involves the transfer of heat energy from one *surface* to another. Drying and increasing humidity around the baby reduces evaporative and transepidermal fluid losses. Increasing air temperature within the incubator may reduce cooling due to convection currents within the incubator, but will not directly reduce radiant heat loss. Clothing or placing a baby in an incubator, or placing an overhead heater to warm the incubator walls, will reduce radiant heat loss.

14. **ABE**

All forms of renal tubular acidosis (RTA) are characterised by a hyperchloraemic metabolic acidosis, with a normal anion gap. In type 1 RTA hypercalciuria and nephrocalcinosis are usual. A typical presentation is with polyuria, polydipsia, failure to thrive and recurrent vomiting. When a metabolic acidosis is present, attempted respiratory compensation is usual, resulting in deep sighing respiration.

15. **BD**

The inflatable portion of the sphygmomanometer cuff should cover at least three-quarters of the length and 40% of the circumference of the upper arm. Sex has no effect on blood pressure in prepubertal children. Blood pressure should be interpreted bearing in mind the child's height centile. If the origin of the left subclavian artery is involved in the coarctation of the aorta, the blood pressure in the *right* arm will be *higher* than the left. Over 80% of hypertension in children has a primary renal cause. An asymptomatic child who is hypertensive does not require immediate treatment. Blood pressure monitoring followed by investigation would be more appropriate.

16. **ABCD**

Tumour lysis syndrome occurs when there is a large tumour load, and massive cell lysis occurs at the start of therapy. Massive cell breakdown is associated with release of intracellular potassium, hyperphosphataemia and hypocalcaemia. Nucleotide breakdown results in the generation of large amounts of uric acid which may crystallise in the renal tubules. The risk of renal sludging and renal failure can be reduced by generous fluid administration, alkalinisation of the urine and administration of allopurinol before starting treatment.

17. **The following physical signs would suggest a neurological lesion at the site stated:**
    A. a hemiplegia and lower motor neurone facial palsy would suggest a pontine lesion.
    B. a hemiplegia with astereognosis would suggest a dominant hemisphere parietal lobe lesion.
    C. mixed upper and lower motor neurone signs in the arms and upper motor neurone signs only in the legs would suggest a cervical cord lesion.
    D. complete loss of vision in the right eye would suggest a right occipital cortex lesion.
    E. loss of shoulder abduction, elbow flexion, forearm pronation and wrist extension would suggest a contralateral internal capsule lesion.

18. **Nutritional rickets is characterised by:**
    A. raised plasma calcium.
    B. raised plasma alkaline phosphatase.
    C. raised plasma phosphate.
    D. raised plasma parathyroid hormone levels.
    E. raised urinary phosphate levels.

19. **The following should be considered with a lower lobe 'pneumonia' which fails to resolve:**
    A. viral pneumonia.
    B. bronchiolitis.
    C. inhaled foreign body.
    D. *Mycobacterium tuberculosis* infection.
    E. congenital abnormality of the lung.

20. **Management of a significant paracetamol ingestion includes:**
    A. immediate intubation and ventilation.
    B. administration of activated charcoal.
    C. forced alkaline diuresis.
    D. administration of *N*-acetylcysteine if indicated by the blood levels.
    E. estimation of the plasma paracetamol level as soon as possible.

**17.  ABC**

A few very simple tests will help to establish the level of the lesion causing a *hemiplegia*. A visual field defect or upper motor neurone facial nerve involvement localises the lesion to the internal capsule or cortex. Lower motor neurone facial nerve involvement locates the lesion within the pons. Cortical dysfunction (e.g. astereognosis) localises the lesion further. Spinal cord lesions usually cause a mixture of upper and lower motor neurone signs at the level of the lesion and upper motor neurone signs below. Blindness in one eye suggests a problem with the eye or optic nerve on that side. The disability described in part E is typical of an Erb's palsy caused by damage to the upper roots (C5 & C6) of the brachial plexus.

**18.  BDE**

In nutritional rickets the diet is deficient in substrate or absorption is impaired. Hypocalcaemia is compensated by secondary hyperparathyroidism which raises calcium levels to normal. Increased bone osteoclastic activity is demonstrated by raised levels of alkaline phosphatase. Parathyroid hormone has a phosphaturic effect, reducing plasma phosphate and increasing urinary phosphate excretion.

**19.  CDE**

Viral pneumonias and bronchiolitis are not usually confined to one lung segment or lobe. A child with a non-resolving pneumonia must have a bronchoscopy to exclude a foreign body. *M. tuberculosis* may cause pneumonia or lobar collapse which will not respond to conventional antibacterials. A congenital lung abnormality, such as a sequestrated lobe, may cause X-ray appearances of a lower lobe consolidation. A sequestrated lobe is a piece of abnormal lung tissue with no normal bronchial or pulmonary vascular connections.

**20.  BD**

Following paracetamol ingestion, there may be no symptoms until liver failure develops up to 5 days later. Activated charcoal will reduce absorption. The paracetamol levels should be measured 4 hours after the ingestion in order to assess the prognosis. For those with a significantly raised paracetamol level *N*-acetylcysteine should be given within 24 hours of the ingestion. Forced diuresis carries a risk of fluid overload.

# 4

# Neurology

1. **These physical signs occur with the CNS lesions described:**
   A. muscle fasciculation and anterior horn cell degeneration.
   B. ataxia and hydrocephalus.
   C. ankle clonus and long-standing cervical spine injury.
   D. athetosis and cerebellar disease.
   E. homonymous hemianopia and unilateral optic nerve damage.

2. **With regard to primitive reflexes, it is abnormal if:**
   A. the Moro reflex persists beyond 2 months of age.
   B. the asymmetric tonic neck reflex (ATNR) is initiated every time the head is turned.
   C. an extensor plantar response is found in a 1-month-old infant.
   D. the grasp reflex of a 3-month-old infant is stronger in the right than left hand.
   E. the rooting reflex is absent at 3 days.

3. **A child can copy:**
   A. a circle by 3 years.
   B. a cross by 4 years.
   C. a straight line by $1\frac{1}{2}$ years.
   D. a triangle by $5\frac{1}{2}$ years.
   E. a square by $3\frac{1}{2}$ years.

4. **The following diagnosis should be considered in the diagnosis of a floppy or hypotonic newborn infant:**
   A. myasthenia gravis.
   B. cervical cord injury following breech delivery.
   C. Werdnig–Hoffman disease (anterior horn cell degeneration).
   D. severe birth asphyxia.
   E. myotonic dystrophy.

1. **ABC**
   Single muscle fibres freed from anterior horn cell control contract independently. Fasciculation may be best seen in the tongue. Ataxia is common in hydrocephalus, particularly if the hydrocephalus involves the 4th ventricle and cerebellum. Hyperreflexia ankle clonus and extensor plantar responses are all typical of long tract damage. Athetosis is usually related to disturbance of basal ganglia function. With unilateral optic nerve damage, reduced visual acuity or blindness in one eye results. A homonymous hemianopia results from unilateral damage to the optic pathways posterior to the optic chiasm.

2. **BDE**
   Developmental or primitive reflexes have usually disappeared by 6 months if not before. Reflexes are abnormal if they are absent, asymmetrical or obligatory (i.e. they can be repeatedly elicited, persist in time such that the infant becomes 'stuck' in the ATNR posture), or persist in time beyond the age of 6 months.

3. **ABD**
   A child can copy a straight line by $2\frac{1}{2}$ years, a circle by 3 years, a cross by 4 years, a square by $4\frac{1}{2}$ years, a triangle by $5\frac{1}{2}$ years and a diamond by 7 years.

4. **ABCDE**
   All of these answers are correct. Myasthenia may be a transient phenomenon if the mother is herself affected or rarely may represent a congenital disease which persists. Cervical cord transection will present as a floppy baby initially, assuming respiration is unaffected, until the period of spinal shock passes when muscle tone increases. In Werdnig–Hoffman disease there is degeneration of the anterior horn cells of the spinal cord, progressive weakness and death after the first 1–2 years of life. Asphyxiated babies in whom muscle tone remains abnormal and who have persistent feeding difficulties have a poor prognosis for normal development. Myotonic dystrophy may present as a profoundly floppy and weak infant who may need respiratory support. The mother is usually affected, though this may have been sufficiently mild to have remained undiagnosed.

5. **The plantar response:**
   A. is elicited by firmly stroking the lateral aspect of the sole.
   B. is normal if extensor in infants under 6 months of age.
   C. is flexor in lower motor neuron lesions of S1,S2 nerve roots.
   D. an extensor response after 1 year of age indicates upper motor neurone pathology.
   E. is absent in infants with extensive thoracic spina bifida.

6. **The following neurological syndromes are characterised by:**
   A. *quadriplegia* – paralysis of all limbs.
   B. *diplegia* – upper-limb rather than lower-limb disability.
   C. *hemiplegia* – proximal muscles more affected than distal muscles.
   D. *hemiplegia* – upper motor neurone lesion affecting arm and leg on one side.
   E. *paraplegia* – lower limbs only affected, upper limbs spared.

7. **Cerebrospinal fluid protein levels are elevated in the following conditions:**
   A. tuberculous meningitis.
   B. Guillain–Barré syndrome.
   C. hypertension.
   D. febrile convulsions.
   E. spinal cord tumour.

8. **Intracranial calcification occurs in at least 50% of patients affected by the following conditions:**
   A. chickenpox.
   B. Sturge–Weber syndrome.
   C. congenital cytomegalovirus encephalitis.
   D. craniopharyngioma.
   E. extradural haematoma.

5. **ABD**

The plantar response tests S1,S2 nerve roots. An extensor plantar response indicates upper motor neurone damage. The plantar response is often equivocal in infancy – an extensor response is definitely abnormal only if occurring spontaneously, is easily elicited and repeatedly extensor, asymmetrical or associated with other abnormal physical signs. With a thoracic myelomeningocele, there will be a segment of isolated cord below the level of the lesion through which unmodified reflex activity takes place and causes extensor responses.

6. **DE**

... plegia indicates a disability of movement and muscle tone and not complete paralysis. Quadriplegia or double hemiplegia indicates that the movement of all four limbs is affected. In a diplegia the proximal muscles of the lower limbs are affected (causing a tendency to scissoring of the legs) more than the upper limbs and is the typical form of cerebral palsy found in ex-preterm infants. In hemiplegias the distal muscles are more markedly affected, producing fisting and toe walking. In a paraplegia only the lower limbs are affected as with spinal cord damage or an interhemispheric lesion.

7. **ABE**

In any condition where there is inflammation or infiltration of the meninges, the CSF protein level will be raised. In Guillain–Barré syndrome there is a demyelinating process in which the CSF protein is characteristically raised but without any increase in CSF cell count. In hypertension and febrile convulsions there is no CNS inflammation and the CSF protein is therefore normal.

8. **BCD**

Intracranial calcification occurs following some intrauterine infections with cytomegalovirus and toxoplasmosis but is uncommon after postnatally acquired infections, with the exception of TB meningitis and cysticercosis. Of the non-infective causes craniopharyngioma, subdural haematoma, A-V malformation and hypo- and pseudohypoparathyroidism are among the commoner causes. In the Sturge–Weber syndrome a capillary naevus over the scalp is associated with an underlying vascular malformation of the meninges and brain which often calcifies.

9. **Neonatal convulsions:**
   A.  will always occur if the blood sugar falls below 2 mmol/L.
   B.  may be associated with maternal hypercalcaemia.
   C.  if focal, would suggest focal pathology.
   D.  should only be investigated if occurring repeatedly.
   E.  have an identifiable cause in around 75% of cases.

10. **Simple febrile convulsions:**
   A.  frequently recur during a 24-hour period.
   B.  may occur at any age between 6 months and 5 years.
   C.  may be focal.
   D.  may sometimes occur without fever.
   E.  should always be investigated by lumbar puncture to exclude meningitis.

11. **Breath-holding attacks:**
   A.  usually occur in association with a high fever.
   B.  may be precipitated by pain.
   C.  may be associated with a short-lasting convulsion.
   D.  may be preceded by crying.
   E.  are associated with asystole.

12. **The following are associated with proptosis:**
   A.  neuroblastoma.
   B.  periorbital cellulitis.
   C.  retinoblastoma.
   D.  craniosynostosis.
   E.  ethmoiditis.

9. **BE**

Neonatal convulsions should be immediately investigated to identify any infection or biochemical disturbance. Hypoglycaemia and hypocalcaemia may cause focal fits in a neonate. Focal fits in older children (over 2–3 years) are more likely to indicate focal pathology. Maternal hyperparathyroidism resulting in hypercalcaemia will cause reversible suppression of fetal parathyroid hormone production, resulting in transient neonatal hypoparathyroidism. There is no absolute level of blood sugar below which fits will occur – in the face of hypoglycaemia, brain functioning is dependent upon the availability of other substrate. Neonatologists prefer to maintain the blood sugar levels above 2.6 mmol/L.

10. **B**

Simple febrile convulsions occur with a high fever and viral infection in children aged between 6 months and 5 years. The fits are short-lasting, generalised and predominantly tonic. Fits usually do not recur during the same illness and are not associated with any neurological abnormality. If a child has fully recovered and a cause for the fever has been identified, then a lumbar puncture is not mandatory.

11. **BCDE**

Breath-holding attacks are often precipitated by anger, frustration or pain. The child may cry briefly, hold his breath, perform a Valsalva manoeuvre and turn blue – i.e. a blue breath-holding attack. Or, usually following a minor injury, he may develop reflex bradycardia or transient asystole – i.e. a reflex anoxic seizure or white breath-holding attack. As with a simple faint, a short-lasting convulsion may occur. Once the child has lost consciousness, breathing returns to normal.

12. **ACDE**

Proptosis either results from a normal eye being pushed forward or from an abnormality within the eye itself. Proptosis may therefore result from retro-orbital tumour (e.g. neuroblastoma), swelling (e.g. orbital cellulitis often associated with an ethmoiditis or cavernous sinus thrombosis), long-standing raised intracranial pressure and/or skull deformity (e.g. craniosynostosis). Tumours within the orbit may also result in proptosis. A periorbital cellulitis involves the superficial tissues of the eyelid anterior to the eye and therefore does not cause proptosis.

13. **Ataxia may be associated with:**
    A. folic acid deficiency.
    B. sedative drugs.
    C. spinal cord dorsal column disease.
    D. cerebellar disease.
    E. marked muscle weakness.

14. **Causes of an acute hemiplegia in a child with congenital heart disease include:**
    A. polycythaemia.
    B. cerebral embolus.
    C. vascular thrombosis.
    D. brain abscess.
    E. migraine.

15. **A 3-year-old suffers an acute left hemiplegia due to a cerebral embolus affecting the right middle meningeal artery. Expected physical signs include:**
    A. aphasia.
    B. deviation of the eyes to the right.
    C. loss of vision in the right eye.
    D. astereognosis of the left hand.
    E. right-sided facial nerve palsy.

16. **Uncontrollable movements may be associated with:**
    A. therapeutic administration of antiemetics.
    B. Streptococcal infection.
    C. neonatal hyperbilirubinaemia.
    D. Duchenne-type muscular dystrophy.
    E. raised serum copper levels.

13. **BCDE**
    Ataxia, or unsteadiness on the feet, may result from: (1) drug or alcohol ingestion; (2) cerebellar disease caused by a tumour, hydrocephalus or infection – chickenpox may be associated with a cerebellaritis; (3) neuropathy affecting afferent or efferent nerves or spinal cord disease; or (4) muscle weakness as in Guillain–Barré syndrome may result in loss of the fine motor control necessary for maintenance of balance.

14. **ABCDE – all of these**
    Increasing polycythaemia is associated with a progressive increase in blood viscosity. Cerebral thrombosis is a recognised complication of congenital cyanotic heart disease, especially if there is polycythaemia, anaemia or dehydration. Cerebral embolus or abscess may complicate cyanotic heart disease. Emboli may complicate arrythmias, cardiac surgery or catheterisation or bacterial endocarditis. Migraine may occur in children with or without cardiac disease and may be complicated by an acute hemiplegia.

15. **BD**
    Left hemisphere dysfunction (right hemiplegia) is associated with speech problems. Loss of vision in the right eye is associated with unilateral retinal or anterior optic nerve dysfunction. A stroke may be associated with a visual field defect if the lesion is above the level of the internal capsule. Eyes deviate towards the side of a cortical lesion. Stereognosis, or the ability to recognise an object placed in the hand, is a function of the contralateral hemisphere. A hemiplegia and crossed facial palsy would suggest that there was pontine involvement.

16. **ABCE**
    Phenothiazines, such as prochlorperazine or metoclopramide, may cause dystonic movements of the eyes, face, neck or trunk – an oculogyric crisis. This is best treated by injection of an anticholinergic drug such as procyclidine. Sydenham's chorea may occur following a group A beta-haemolytic Streptococcal infection. Chorea, an extrapyramidal tract disorder, also occurs in Wilson's disease where there is an abnormality in copper metabolism and in kernicterus caused by bilirubin damage to the basal ganglia. Movements are simply weak in Duchenne muscular dystrophy.

17. **The following would be typical of a febrile convulsion:**
    A. duration of more than 15 minutes.
    B. occurrence in a female less than 5 months old.
    C. postictal Todd's paralysis.
    D. fever not > 38°C over the next 24 hours.
    E. a family history of febrile seizures in 40% of cases.

18. **The risk of epilepsy after a single febrile convulsion:**
    A. is approximately 5–10%.
    B. is increased if there is a family history of febrile fits.
    C. is increased if there is a family history of afebrile fits.
    D. is increased if the convulsion was focal in nature.
    E. is increased if the convulsion was prolonged – i.e. over 30 minutes.

19. **Causes of a unilateral constricted pupil include:**
    A. Horner syndrome.
    B. 3rd nerve palsy.
    C. optic nerve tumour.
    D. barbiturate ingestion.
    E. retinopathy of prematurity.

20. **Ptosis occurs:**
    A. as a congenital variant.
    B. as a result of a facial nerve palsy.
    C. as a result of a 5th cranial nerve palsy.
    D. as a result of a Horner syndrome.
    E. as a result of a 3rd nerve palsy.

**17.  E**

Febrile fits are short, associated with a high fever and are generalised. There is no postictal neurological abnormality. Fits tend not to recur during the same illness. There is a strong family history (40%) and autosomal dominant inheritance is suggested by the pattern of attack in some families. Typically, children between 6 months and 5 years are affected.

**18.  CDE**

In otherwise normal children, the risk of epilepsy after a simple febrile seizure is no greater than the average population – i.e. around 1%. A family history of *afebrile* fits is associated with an increased risk of epilepsy. Any atypical convulsion with fever is associated with a subsequently greater risk of epilepsy.

**19.  A**

A Horner syndrome causes a small pupil, ptosis, facial anhidrosis and enophthalmos due to damage to the sympathetic fibres to the eye. A 3rd nerve palsy may be associated with loss of parasympathetic fibres leading to unopposed sympathetic action – i.e. a dilated pupil and an eye turned down and out. An optic nerve tumour and retinopathy of prematurity will not of themselves cause any abnormality of pupillary size, though pupillary reflexes may be affected if the optic nerve or retina are severely damaged. Opiates and barbiturates may cause pupillary constriction, but not unilateral.

**20.  ADE**

Ptosis may result from weakness of the levator palpebrae muscle or abnormality in its innervation. There may be a congenital abnormality of the levator muscle, weakness due to myasthenia or muscular dystrophy or abnormality of innervation, as part of a Horner syndrome or 3rd nerve palsy.

21. **The following anticonvulsant treatment would be appropriate:**
    A. phenytoin as first choice for temporal lobe seizures.
    B. sodium valproate for primary generalised tonic/clonic seizures.
    C. prednisolone for infantile spasms.
    D. phenobarbitone for frequent, recurrent febrile seizures.
    E. carbamazepine for recurrent hypoglycaemic convulsions.

22. **Recognised side-effects of certain anticonvulsants include:**
    A. hyperactivity and phenobarbitone.
    B. gum hypertrophy and carbamazepine.
    C. acute liver toxicity and sodium valproate.
    D. rickets and phenytoin.
    E. rage and carbamazepine.

23. **Management of status epilepticus should include:**
    A. intramuscular diazepam immediately on arrival in hospital.
    B. low-concentration oxygen if there is any respiratory difficulty.
    C. sedation with a short-acting barbiturate if the patient remains agitated after the seizure has been terminated.
    D. intravenous phenytoin if appropriate initial therapy is ineffective.
    E. generous rehydration fluid administration.

24. **Problems which may arise as a result of a prolonged seizure include:**
    A. respiratory alkalosis.
    B. metabolic acidosis.
    C. hypokalaemia.
    D. aspiration pneumonia.
    E. raised intracranial pressure.

**21. BC**

Principles of anticonvulsant therapy in children include: sodium valproate for the genetic seizure disorders – simple absence seizures ('petit mal'), generalised tonic/clonic, myoclonic seizures and febrile convulsions. Carbamazepine (phenytoin, lamotrogine or sodium valproate) for the lesional epilepsies related to structural abnormalities. ACTH, prednisolone, benzodiazepines, vigabatrin, phenobarbitone or pyridoxine for the malignant epilepsy syndromes such as infantile spasms and Lennox Gastaut. Fits due to hypoglycaemia require the cause to be determined – treatment is with dextrose.

**22. ACD**

Gum hypertrophy is a side-effect of phenytoin and cyclosporin therapy. In young children phenobarbitone may cause a paradoxical hyperactivity. Acute liver toxicity and hepatic failure are rare side-effects of sodium valproate. Liver function tests should be checked before and after starting valproate therapy. Phenytoin may cause biochemical rickets after prolonged therapy. Rage may be a feature of temporal lobe epilepsy, and may be treated with carbamazepine.

**23. D**

Diazepam should be given intravenously (IV) or rectally for treatment of status epilepticus. Sufficient oxygen should be given to correct hypoxia; there is no risk of respiratory depression from high oxygen concentration in acutely ill children. There is no place for sedation of the postictal child. Continuing irritability may be due to cerebral oedema, continuing subclinical fits or CNS infection. Intravenous phenytoin is indicated if fits have not been effectively treated with diazepam or paraldehyde. The risk of cerebral oedema is reduced by restricting fluids after a prolonged convulsion.

**24. BDE**

A combined metabolic (lactic) and respiratory acidosis is the usual blood gas abnormality after a prolonged convulsion. Hyperkalaemia may develop acutely in the face of an acidosis (potassium leaks out of the cells). Aspiration of vomit may occur while unconscious. Raised intracranial pressure may occur as a result of a deficiency in cerebral oxygenation and substrate delivery during a prolonged fit.

25. **Focal seizures are:**
    A. indicative of focal pathology.
    B. associated with a preceding aura.
    C. are not accompanied by loss of consciousness.
    D. associated with transient paralysis.
    E. reliably diagnosed if a seizure is witnessed from the onset.

26. **In a child with focal seizures the following clinical features would suggest the underlying diagnosis:**
    A. a left hemiplegia.
    B. macrocephaly.
    C. depigmented patches over the skin.
    D. intracranial bruit.
    E. unilateral cataract.

27. **Temporal lobe epilepsy:**
    A. is characterised by a 3/s spike and wave EEG abnormality.
    B. is associated with prolonged convulsions in earlier child-hood.
    C. is best treated with phenytoin.
    D. is characterised by generalised tonic/clonic seizure activity.
    E. may be associated with an homonymous visual field defect.

28. **'Petit mal' epilepsy (simple absence seizures):**
    A. is often associated with poor school performance.
    B. is a lifelong condition.
    C. is characterised by lip smacking and/or repetitive hand movements.
    D. is effectively treated with ethosuxamide.
    E. occurs only in the prepubertal child.

**25.  BD**

In children under 3 years of age a focal fit does not necessarily indicate focal pathology. Focal fits (e.g. temporal lobe fits) may be preceded by an aura. The seizure activity may undergo rapid generalisation, so that a generalised fit develops. This transition may be so rapid that even a trained observer may be unaware of the focal nature of the onset of the fit. A transient paralysis/ aphasia/sensory disturbance may follow a focal seizure.

**26.  ACD**

A hemiplegia indicates unilateral cortical pathology, depigmented patches over the skin suggest tuberose sclerosis and an intracranial bruit suggests an A-V malformation – all suggestive of an underlying structural brain lesion which may be a focus for seizure activity. Macrocephaly is suggestive of a generalised disorder of brain growth and/or development. Unilateral cataract is not suggestive of any disease causing focal seizures.

**27.  BE**

Temporal lobe epilepsy is suggested by an aura prior to the seizure, followed by some of the following features: automatic movements, repetitive movements and lack of awareness. There is amnesia for the event. The seizure may become generalised. An EEG may demonstrate temporal lobe spike activity. The optic radiation's course through the temporal lobe and a structural lesion here may cause a homonymous superior quadrantanopsia.

**28.  ADE**

Simple absence ('petit mal') epilepsy is one of the genetic epilepsies and commonly behaves as an autosomal dominant trait. It is characterised by a very stereotyped 3/s spike and wave abnormality on the EEG. It occurs in children aged 3–12 years and is not associated with any automatic movements. A brief absence without loss of posture occurs. There is no awareness of the event which may occur, in some cases, many times during the day, which results in loss of ability to concentrate and maintain a train of thought. It is therefore an important diagnosis to consider in a child whose school performance is deteriorating. The absences may be brought on by over-breathing.

29. **Infantile spasms:**
    A. usually occur between 1 and 4 years of age.
    B. may be confused with infantile colic.
    C. are exclusively extensor in nature.
    D. are associated with subsequent developmental delay in the majority of cases.
    E. have an identifiable underlying cause in less than 10% of cases.

30. **The following are examples of primary generalised seizures:**
    A. temporal lobe epilepsy.
    B. akinetic seizures – drop attacks.
    C. infantile spasms.
    D. 'petit mal' epilepsy.
    E. benign Rolandic epilepsy.

31. **Hydrocephalus:**
    A. is suggested by transillumination of the skull.
    B. is best diagnosed in neonates by magnetic resonance imaging.
    C. is associated with microcephaly.
    D. is more commonly of communicating than non-communicating type.
    E. is always present in infants with spina bifida.

32. **Early signs and symptoms of raised intracranial pressure in a 6-month-old infant include:**
    A. increased appetite.
    B. irritability.
    C. papilloedema.
    D. separation of the coronal sutures.
    E. loss of upward gaze.

**29.   BD**
Infantile spasms occur predominantly in the 4 to 9 months age group. The seizures consist of flexion of the arms, neck and legs and a cry is sometimes emitted. This may cause the fits to be mistaken for infantile colic. Occasionally the seizures may have an extensor component of the arms as in a Moro response. Approximately 40% of infantile spasms are idiopathic and these infants have a 50% chance of recovery and normal development. The majority have a pre-existing abnormality of brain development or biochemistry and have a poor prognosis.

**30.   BCD**
Temporal lobe epilepsy and benign Rolandic epilepsy are focal epilepsies, though the seizure discharge may become generalised. The others are generalised seizure disorders, with generalised EEG abnormality.

**31.   AD**
Transillumination of the skull (the head lights up like a Chinese lantern) is suggestive of gross hydrocephalus or hydranencephalus. Before closure of the anterior fontanelle, ventricular size is most easily imaged with ultrasound. Hydrocephalus is usually associated with an enlarged head, which increases in size faster than normal after birth, unless the hydrocephalus has 'arrested'. Hydrocephalus is more commonly communicating, though this terminology is now falling out of favour. Infants with a myelomeningocele usually have hydrocephalus. The term spina bifida includes 'occulta', meningocele and myelomeningocele. Hydrocephalus is not always present in all of these lesions.

**32.   BD**
Early signs and symptoms of raised intracranial pressure (ICP) in infants with open sutures include a disproportionately rapid increase in head circumference. This may be accompanied by separation of the cranial sutures. Irritability and drowsiness with a tendency to repeated vomiting are early signs of raised ICP. Loss of conjugate upward gaze due to raised pressure in the 4th ventricle is a late sign. Papilloedema in infants may not occur unless the ICP rises very quickly as separation of the sutures may prevent markedly raised ICP.

33. **Cerebrospinal fluid:**
    A. is mainly formed by drainage of brain interstitial fluid into the ventricle.
    B. flows from the lateral ventricle into the 3rd ventricle via the aqueduct of Sylvius.
    C. protein levels are equivalent to plasma levels.
    D. glucose levels are equivalent to plasma levels.
    E. normally contains up to $100 \times 10^6/L$ white cells.

34. **A subdural haematoma:**
    A. is associated with the shaken baby syndrome.
    B. presents with microcephaly.
    C. is associated with fits.
    D. may progressively increase in size over time.
    E. is best treated with a ventriculo-peritoneal shunt.

35. **Cerebral palsy is:**
    A. caused by intrapartum asphyxia in most cases.
    B. characterised by both motor and sensory abnormalities.
    C. a condition for life – one does not 'outgrow' cerebral palsy.
    D. associated with progressive dementia.
    E. associated with an increased risk of fits.

36. **Signs of increased muscle tone in the lower limbs, extensor plantar responses and ankle clonus would be compatible with a diagnosis of:**
    A. acute poliomyelitis.
    B. diplegia of prematurity.
    C. Duchenne muscular dystrophy.
    D. spinal cord tumour.
    E. thoracic myelomeningocele.

**33. None of these**

Cerebrospinal fluid (CSF) is formed by the choroid plexus and flows from the lateral ventricles into the 3rd ventricle and then through the aqueduct of Sylvius into the 4th ventricle. Normal CSF protein values of 0.2–0.4 g/L compare with total plasma protein level of 60–80 g/L. CSF glucose values should be 50–60% of the plasma value. Normal CSF outside the newborn period contains $5–10 \times 10^6/L$ white blood cells.

**34. ACD**

A subdural haematoma forms as a result of rupture of bridging veins in the potential subdural space. As the clot liquefies leakage of albumen and fluid into the space causes further enlargement. Subdural haematoma is a common aftermath of a shaking injury to an infant. Acceleration and deceleration injuries (and sometimes skull impact injuries) also commonly occur. Seizures and a rapidly enlarging head are typical presenting signs. Ventriculo-peritoneal shunt is a treatment for *hydrocephalus* with enlargement of the ventricles. Aspiration and drainage of the subdural fluid may allow resolution. A 'subdural-peritoneal' shunt may be performed for chronic subdurals which do not resolve with simple treatment.

**35. E**

By definition, cerebral palsy (CP) is a non-progressive disorder of *movement* or posture – sensory disturbance is not an essential component of the condition, although disturbances of sensation are common, especially in the more severely affected children. Intrapartum asphyxia may account for only 20% of CP. In one study 55% of infants diagnosed as having CP at 1 year had no evidence of CP at 7 years. Fits are a common accompaniment of CP.

**36. BDE**

The signs described here are those of an upper motor neurone lesion affecting the legs, as in a spinal cord lesion or diplegia. In poliomyelitis there is anterior horn cell disease and flaccid paralysis of the lower limbs. If there is an isolated segment of cord below the level of a neural tube defect, there will be uninhibited reflex activity and upper motor neurone signs as described.

37. **A congenital hemiplegia:**
    A. is the commonest form of cerebral palsy related to prematurity.
    B. may present with early development of hand preference.
    C. usually prevents independent walking.
    D. is characterised by a greater increase in distal (rather than proximal) muscle tone.
    E. is associated with ipsilateral muscle wasting.

38. **The head circumference of a 6-month-old infant lies 1 cm above the 97th percentile. Causes for this finding include:**
    A. hydrocephalus.
    B. Down syndrome.
    C. fetal alcohol syndrome.
    D. familial macrocephaly.
    E. normal baby.

39. **Causes of microcephaly include:**
    A. hydranencephaly.
    B. phenylketonuria.
    C. trisomy 18.
    D. craniosynostosis.
    E. severe birth asphyxia.

40. **Progressive dementia may be causally associated with:**
    A. neonatal kernicterus.
    B. severe birth asphyxia.
    C. hypothyroidism.
    D. Down syndrome.
    E. measles infection earlier in childhood.

### 37. BDE

Diplegia is the commonest form of neurological abnormality related to prematurity. Hand preference developing before 18 months should always raise the possibility of a problem with the least preferred hand. A hemiplegia alone rarely prevents walking. Walking may be difficult due to problems with 'swing-through' of the foot. Predominantly increased distal muscle tone is characteristic of a hemiplegia. A hemiplegic limb may be wasted and shorter than the normal limb.

### 38. ADE

A single measurement of the head circumference which plots above the 97th percentile is not significant unless associated with other abnormal findings suggestive of raised ICP. Familial macrocephaly is common. Babies with Down syndrome and fetal alcohol syndrome tend to have relatively small heads even in proportion to the rest of their body, which also tends to be small.

### 39. BCDE

Hydranencephaly causes a large fluid-filled head which transilluminates with a bright light. The usual cause of microcephaly is poor brain growth. Phenylalanine in high concentration is toxic to the developing brain and can cause microcephaly in children with PKU or in the fetuses of mothers who themselves have PKU, unless plasma phenylalanine levels are carefully controlled by diet during pregnancy. A severely damaged or intrinsically abnormal brain will fail to grow normally. Premature fusion of the cranial sutures usually occurs due to poor brain growth. Occasionally this may happen while normal brain growth is continuing and raised intracranial pressure may result.

### 40. DE

Neonatal kernicterus and birth asphyxia cause a non-progressive brain damage. Intelligence may or may not be affected. Down syndrome is associated with premature dementia. Measles infection is associated with later development of subacute sclerosing panencephalitis, characterised by personality change, loss of skills, myoclonic jerks and progressive neurological deterioration. Hypothyroidism if undiagnosed is associated with delayed development or deteriorating school performance, but not irreversible loss of skills already acquired.

41. **The following are present in the stated causes of dementia:**
    A. papilloedema in the leukodystrophies.
    B. hypoglycaemia in mucopolysaccharidosis type 1 – Hurler syndrome.
    C. hepatosplenomegaly in phenylketonuria.
    D. corneal clouding in glycogen storage disease type 1.
    E. cherry red spot in Tay–Sachs disease.

42. **In a comatose child:**
    A. a posture with the arms flexed at the elbows indicates bilateral hemisphere damage.
    B. reactive pupils indicates an intact midbrain.
    C. a unilateral fixed and dilated pupil indicates an ipsilateral 6th cranial nerve palsy.
    D. a posture with extension of the arms and legs indicates an upper brainstem lesion.
    E. absence of the corneal reflex is suggestive of a pontine lesion.

43. **Causes of sudden-onset coma include:**
    A. hypothyroidism.
    B. ventricular fibrillation.
    C. paracetamol poisoning.
    D. hypoglycaemia.
    E. epilepsy.

44. **Initial management of an unconscious, febrile, 4-year-old child in the A&E department should include:**
    A. administration of empirical intravenous anticonvulsant.
    B. estimation of blood gases.
    C. estimation of blood sugar.
    D. lumbar puncture.
    E. intravenous fluids at 150 ml/kg/day.

**41.  E.**
Optic atrophy and brain atrophy are likely to occur in the leukodystrophies. Hypoglycaemia is not a feature of any of the mucopolysaccharidoses in which mucopolysaccharide is laid down in tissues. Very high plasma phenylalanine levels cause CNS toxicity but without storage of abnormal metabolites. Glycogen storage diseases do not cause corneal opacity – this is a common feature of Hurler syndrome. Hypoglycaemia occurs in some of the forms of glycogen storage disease, including glucose-6-phosphatase deficiency.

**42.  ABDE**
Decorticate posturing – elbows flexed – is suggestive of bilateral damage above the level of the brainstem. Decerebrate posturing with arms and legs extended is suggestive of deeper damage to hemispheres or upper brainstem. Reactive pupils imply an intact midbrain. Absent corneal reflex suggests a pontine lesion or dysfunction as in poisoning. A unilateral fixed and dilated pupil is suggestive of a 3rd nerve lesion, as may occur in a tentorial herniation, due to raised supratentorial pressure.

**43.  DE**
Hypothyroidism is associated with insidious onset of symptoms. Ventricular fibrillation is rare in children and is a cause of sudden death, not coma. Serious paracetamol poisoning usually causes symptoms of liver toxicity 3–5 days after ingestion. Hypoglycaemia and seizures are important causes of coma. All comatose or drowsy children should have an immediate blood sugar measurement.

**44.  BC**
Anticonvulsants should not be given unless there is clinical evidence of continuing seizure activity. Blood gas measurement will give important information about gas exchange and pH balance for both management and diagnosis. Blood sugar estimation is vital, and if less than 3 mmol/L, further blood samples should be drawn and intravenous dextrose given immediately afterwards. Lumbar puncture should not be performed if raised ICP is possible. Intravenous fluids should be restricted to two-thirds normal maintenance if there is any possibility of raised ICP.

**45. Headache:**
   A. associated with a stiff neck is diagnostic of meningitis.
   B. without papilloedema excludes raised intracranial pressure.
   C. associated with vomiting is diagnostic of raised intracranial pressure.
   D. associated with an intracranial bruit indicates the presence of an arteriovenous malformation.
   E. in a 4-year-old is most likely to be due to anxiety.

**46. Features more typical of migraine than tension headaches include:**
   A. associated lightheadedness.
   B. insomnia.
   C. headache causing waking from sleep.
   D. constant pain over several weeks.
   E. generalised headache.

**47. Migraine:**
   A. is usually associated with nausea or vomiting.
   B. does not occur in children under 6 years.
   C. is characterised by the headache consistently affecting the same side of the head.
   D. may be complicated by a transient loss of speech.
   E. does not affect the EEG.

**48. Recognised precipitants of migraine include:**
   A. stress.
   B. Coca-Cola.
   C. exercise.
   D. cheese.
   E. chocolate.

**45.  None of these**

Headache with neck stiffness could indicate meningitis but could equally well indicate raised intracranial pressure. Papilloedema is a very unreliable sign of raised ICP in children. Headache and vomiting is compatible with but certainly not diagnostic of raised ICP: a viral infection is statistically very much more likely. Altered level of consciousness is by far the most important sign of raised ICP. Intracranial bruits in young children are frequently heard and, although present with intracranial A-V malformations, may also be heard with raised ICP or in conditions producing a hyperdynamic circulation as in fever or anaemia. Headache in young children is not a common symptom and is unlikely to be due to anxiety.

**46.  C**

Migraine may be associated with true vertigo, nausea, vomiting and photophobia. Headaches may come in clusters with symptom-free intervals. Migraine headaches may cause waking from sleep. Migraine headaches are usually bifrontal, occipital or classically one-sided. Lightheadedness, insomnia, prolonged unremitting headaches and generalised headaches are *more likely* to be related to anxiety than migraine.

**47.  AD**

Migraine is usually associated with nausea or sickness. In young children gastrointestinal symptoms predominate – i.e. abdominal migraine. Headache tends to occur in older children. Headache always affecting the same side of the head is not typical of migraine (only 20% in one study) and should raise suspicion of an alternative diagnosis. Migraine may be complicated by hemiparesis, aphasia, ophthalmoplegia, visual or sensory disturbance or fits. The EEG is frequently abnormal during an attack.

**48.  ABCDE – all of these**

A wide variety of triggers may be responsible for migraine in those who are predisposed. Dietary triggers are uncommon in childhood.

**49. A child with a mid-thoracic myelomeningocele will:**
   A. have normal hand function.
   B. have a flaccid paralysis of both legs.
   C. be at risk of developing a progressive restrictive ventilation defect.
   D. be at risk of reflux nephropathy.
   E. have sensory loss below the level of the lesion.

**50. Signs of early posterior spinal cord compression include:**
   A. foot drop.
   B. ankle clonus.
   C. extensor plantar responses.
   D. loss of vibration sense in the feet.
   E. urinary retention.

**51. Conditions associated with spinal cord compression include:**
   A. neurofibromatosis.
   B. cystic fibrosis.
   C. Down syndrome.
   D. achondroplasia.
   E. neuroblastoma.

**52. Long-term problems following an acquired thoracic spinal cord transection include:**
   A. pressure sores.
   B. reflux nephropathy.
   C. hydrocephalus.
   D. progressive joint contractures of the lower limbs.
   E. 'phantom limb' pain.

**49.   CDE**

Hand function is commonly abnormal in children with hydrocephalus as a result of ventricular dilatation damaging cortical fibres and poor cerebellar function. If there is a segment of undamaged spinal cord below the level of the lesion, then unmodified reflex activity can take place and the lower limbs may be hypertonic as a result. The same mechanism may result in uncoordinated activity of the bladder detrusor and sphincter muscles. High pressure generated in the bladder may result in vesico-ureteric reflux. Mid-thoracic paralysis with or without hemivertebrae commonly leads to a progressive scoliosis with resultant restrictive ventilation defect. There will be anaesthesia below the level of the lesion.

**50.   D**

Foot drop and urinary retention are late signs of cord compression. Ankle clonus is a clear sign of increased muscle tone and will appear relatively late. Plantar responses may be flexor and reflexes reduced in the early stages. The posterior columns may be affected early causing loss of vibration sense.

**51.   ACDE**

Intraspinal neuromas may cause cord compression and paraplegia in neurofibromatosis. Down syndrome children are at increased risk of atlanto-axial dislocation. In achondroplasia there may be brainstem compression due to narrowing of the foramen magnum and a narrow spinal canal may cause cord compression. Metastases from neuroblastoma to the spine may cause cord compression. There is no reason for cystic fibrosis to cause cord problems.

**52.   ABD**

Thoracic cord transection will cause complete loss of sensation below the level of the lesion. Skin ischaemia resulting from the body weight or friction from ill-fitting shoes or splints will pass unnoticed and skin breakdown may result. Reflex activity in the cord below the level of the lesion may result in uncoordinated action of the bladder detrusor and sphincter muscle, leading to high-pressure vesico-ureteric reflux. The unequal strength of unregulated, opposing muscle groups may cause progressive joint deformity. There is no reason for hydrocephalus or 'phantom limb' pain to develop in this situation.

53. **Modest hyperreflexia to the knee jerk reflex is likely to be abnormal if:**
    A. there is associated ipsilateral muscle hypertrophy.
    B. there is associated crossed adductor activity.
    C. the hyperreflexia is unilateral.
    D. the reflex can be elicited by tapping over the mid-tibia.
    E. there is an associated flexor plantar response.

54. **Clinical features of significance in diagnosing the cause of symmetrical lower-limb hyperreflexia in an alert 4-year-old would include:**
    A. axillary freckles.
    B. multiple depigmented skin patches.
    C. lipoma in the lumbar region.
    D. flexural eczema
    E. papilloedema.

55. **A 5-year-old boy presents with a 2-week history of a flu-like illness followed by a persistent cough. One day before admission he becomes unsteady on his feet and has difficulty going upstairs. On examination he appears well, has no respiratory distress and is alert and fully cooperative. There is normal power in the upper limbs and grade 3/6 power in the lower limbs. Reflexes are absent in the legs. Plantar responses are flexor. CXR shows patchy change:**
    A. the apparent muscle weakness is probably hysterical.
    B. a sensory level will be detectable on careful neurological examination.
    C. a lumbar puncture is likely to be dangerous.
    D. the muscle weakness is unlikely to progress.
    E. the respiratory infection is coincidental and not associated with the presenting clinical problem.

56. **In the case outlined above:**
    A. there is likely to be a CSF lymphocytosis.
    B. peripheral nerve conduction studies will be normal.
    C. repeated monitoring of the vital capacity is necessary.
    D. the parents should be advised that a full recovery is expected.
    E. cardiac arrhythmias may occur.

**53. BCD**

Reflexes are likely to be abnormal if: (1) asymmetrical; (2) exaggerated in amplitude; (3) there is a wide afferent field – i.e. if the reflex can be elicited away from the usual point of stimulus; and (4) there are crossed responses. An extensor plantar response and muscle wasting might be associated with abnormally brisk reflexes.

**54. ACE**

Bilateral hyperreflexia of the lower limbs may result from raised ICP, frontal tumour or a spinal cord lesion. Axillary freckling and pigmented skin lesions are features of neurofibromatosis type 1 in which there may be spinal cord compression. Depigmented skin lesions could indicate a diagnosis of tuberose sclerosis, but this is not associated with cord problems. A lumbar lipoma could be associated with an underlying lipoma of the cord and may be an important sign. Eczema would not be relevant. Papilloedema could be due to a slowly growing intracranial tumour which could result in hyperreflexia.

**55. None of these**

This boy has classical Guillain–Barré disease. This is a condition classically associated with a progressive ascending muscle weakness which may occasionally affect the autonomic nervous system and may cause respiratory muscle weakness and a bulbar palsy. Sensory abnormalities may occur, but a sensory level as seen in cord damage will not be present. The diagnosis is confirmed by finding an acellular CSF and raised CSF protein level. The preceding respiratory infection is common. This boy may have had a mycoplasma infection.

**56. CDE**

The CSF should be acellular. There is peripheral nerve conduction abnormality; this condition is a parainfectious demyelinating polyneuritis. Respiratory failure, due to weakness of the respiratory muscles, is a real possibility and careful monitoring of the vital capacity or other easily repeated assessment of maximal ventilation is important. As a part of the autonomic nervous system dysfunction hypertension or cardiac arrythmias may occur. A full recovery is to be expected.

57. **The following are highly suggestive of the diagnosis given in an infant presenting with altered conscious level:**
    A. retinal haemorrhages and shaking injury.
    B. ingestion of therapeutic doses of aspirin for fever and Reye syndrome.
    C. respiratory alkalosis and hyperammoniaemia.
    D. intracranial bruit and an arteriovenous malformation.
    E. ketotic hypoglycaemia and deliberate insulin poisoning.

58. **The following muscles are innervated by the nerve roots indicated:**
    A. deltoid muscle – C5 nerve root.
    B. biceps muscle – T5 nerve root.
    C. small muscles of the hand – T1 nerve root.
    D. quadriceps muscle – L2 nerve root.
    E. extraocular muscles of the eye – C1 nerve root.

59. **Loss of sensation in the following areas results from damage to the nerve or nerve roots indicated:**
    A. back of the hand – knuckles of 2nd and 3rd fingers – C5 & C6.
    B. cornea – facial nerve.
    C. perianal region – S1 & S2.
    D. dorsum of the foot – L5.
    E. back of the head – trigeminal nerve.

60. **An Erb palsy found on routine neonatal examination:**
    A. is more likely to occur in low birth weight infants than those with birth weight over 4 kg.
    B. results from damage to the lower roots of the brachial plexus.
    C. results in weakness of the deltoid and brachioradialis muscles.
    D. results in loss of the grasp reflex of the affected hand.
    E. is usually associated with an ipsilateral Horner syndrome.

57. **ABCD**

   Haemorrhage from the retinal veins occurs when there has been a rapid increase in venous pressure, typically as a result of a shaking injury with squeezing of the chest. Aspirin should not be given to febrile children as it may cause Reye syndrome, an illness characterised by dysfunction of the mitochondria, fatty infiltration of the liver, liver cell dysfunction and brain swelling. A respiratory alkalosis is associated with hyperammoniaemia, probably as a result of a mild degree of cerebral oedema causing hyperventilation. An intracranial bruit may be related both to raised ICP and flow through an A-V malformation. When hypoglycaemia results from hyperinsulinism, there should be no ketones in the urine as fat metabolism should be effectively switched off by the effect of insulin forcing glucose into the cells.

58. **ACD**

   Deltoid – C5; biceps – C6; hand muscles – T1.
   Quadriceps – L2; eye – cranial nerves 3, 4 & 6.

59. **AD**

   The radial side of the dorsum of the hand is innervated by the radial nerve – C5–8. Sensory fibres to the cornea are supplied by the trigeminal nerve. The perianal region is innervated by S4 & 5. The dorsum of the foot is innervated by L5 & S1. The back of the head is innervated by C2 & C3.

60. **C**

   Birth trauma is more common in large babies than small and preterm babies. The upper roots of the brachial plexus are damaged usually by overextension of the neck in an effort to deliver the anterior shoulder. C5 & 6 damage causes weakness of deltoid, biceps, brachioradialis and the extensor muscles of the forearm – i.e. an Erb palsy. The small muscles of the hand are unaffected. Horner syndrome is found in 30% of babies affected by Klumpke paralysis in which the lower nerve roots of the brachial plexus are damaged.

61. **A facial nerve palsy – a Bell's palsy – is associated with:**
    A. an inability to open the eye on the affected side.
    B. loss of movement of the whole of the face on the affected side.
    C. preservation of movement associated with emotion (e.g. crying).
    D. loss of tear production on the affected side.
    E. loss of sensation over the anterior two-thirds of the tongue.

62. **A facial nerve palsy is associated with:**
    A. myotonic dystrophy.
    B. mumps.
    C. Guillain–Barré syndrome.
    D. glioma of the medulla oblongata.
    E. hypertension.

63. **Primary brain tumours in children over 1 year of age:**
    A. are mostly supratentorial.
    B. form the commonest type of solid tumour in this age group.
    C. usually present with focal seizures.
    D. often present with ataxia.
    E. metastasise to the lungs.

64. **The following brain tumours and features have a recognised association:**
    A. craniopharyngioma and suprasellar calcification on skull X-ray.
    B. astrocytoma and multiple CNS metastases.
    C. pontine glioma and cranial nerve palsies with pyramidal tract signs.
    D. optic nerve glioma and optic atrophy.
    E. medulloblastoma and ataxia.

**61. B**

A facial nerve palsy causes an inability to *close* the eye, thus putting the cornea at risk of damage from drying. An upper motor neuron facial nerve lesion results in weakness of the facial muscles, but with relative sparing of the upper part of the face. A Bell's palsy affects both upper and lower parts of the face and does not allow movement with emotion. Tear production continues and may overflow from the drooping lower lid. The petrosal nerve and chorda tympani are branches of the facial nerve which are not usually involved in a Bell's palsy. The petrosal nerve supplies the lacrimal glands. The chorda tympani is motor to the submandibular and sublingual glands and is sensory to the anterior two-thirds of the tongue.

**62. BCE**

In myotonic dystrophy there is an expressionless face due to weakness of the facial muscles and not due to a facial nerve palsy. Mumps, Guillain–Barré syndrome and hypertension are all associated with facial nerve palsies but a medullary glioma will not affect the facial nerve which arises in the pons.

**63. BD**

Brain tumours in young children are predominantly infratentorial. As a group, brain tumours are the commonest form of solid tumour in childhood. As most tumours are infratentorial, these tumours usually present with posterior fossa and/or brainstem symptoms such as ataxia, vomiting, hydrocephalus, diplopia, stiff neck and/or pyramidal tract signs. Fits and hemiparesis are a feature of *supra*tentorial tumours. Brain tumours usually spread only within the CNS.

**64. ACDE**

Calcification above the pituitary fossa is one of the characteristics of craniopharyngioma. There may be visual field defects, growth problems and symptoms of raised intracranial pressure. An astrocytoma is relatively benign and does not invade or metastasise. Cranial nerve palsies and long tract signs without raised intracranial pressure are diagnostic of a brainstem tumour, usually a glioma. An optic nerve glioma may present with decreased visual acuity and either papilloedema or optic nerve atrophy, usually at a later stage. As noted above, posterior fossa tumours – e.g. medulloblastoma – commonly present with ataxia.

65. **Lumbar puncture is mandatory to exclude meningitis:**
    A. whenever there is headache and neck stiffness.
    B. after a convulsion in a febrile 18-month-old.
    C. in a child with a typical rash of meningococcal septicaemia.
    D. in any child with an altered level of consciousness.
    E. in all children who have sustained a skull fracture.

66. **In the UK organisms commonly causing meningitis in a 2-year-old child include:**
    A. *E. coli.*
    B. *H. influenzae.*
    C. Group B *beta*-haemolytic Streptococci.
    D. *Streptococcus pneumoniae.*
    E. *Listeria monocytogenes.*

67. **Complications of acute bacterial meningitis include:**
    A. inappropriate antidiuretic hormone secretion.
    B. hypoglycaemia.
    C. convulsions.
    D. cranial nerve palsies.
    E. intracranial haemorrhage.

68. **A blocked ventriculo-peritoneal shunt would be suggested by:**
    A. irritability.
    B. drowsiness.
    C. vomiting.
    D. a bruit over the anterior fontanelle.
    E. absent diastolic flow on Doppler recording of cerebral blood flow.

**65. None of these**

Lumbar puncture (LP) is never mandatory. An LP should not be carried out if there is any alteration of conscious level. Even in suspected meningitis, it may be safer to begin treatment and for an LP to be carried out later. Headache and neck stiffness are symptoms which are suggestive not only of meningitis, but also of raised intracranial pressure or a posterior fossa tumour. In meningococcal septicaemia treatment is unchanged if meningitis is diagnosed. The risk of death from coning is increased if an LP is performed. Most febrile infants who have had a convulsion will have had a simple febrile fit. If the child makes a complete recovery, there is no need for an LP. There is no place for an LP in the routine management of children with skull fractures.

**66. D**

*E. coli*, Group B Streptococcus and Listeria are recognised causes of neonatal meningitis but are uncommon in older children. *Haemophilus meningitis* is now rare since routine Hib vaccine in the 1st year of life. Meningococcal and Pneumococcal meningitis are now the two commonest bacteria causing meningitis in otherwise healthy infants and toddlers.

**67. ACD**

Any condition causing brain swelling may cause inappropriate ADH secretion. Hypoglycaemia and intracranial haemorrhage would be unexpected outside the neonatal period. Seizures are common (30%) in bacterial meningitis. Cranial nerve palsies are seen especially in basal meningitis.

**68. All of these**

Infants with a blocked ventriculo-peritoneal (VP) shunt develop effortless vomiting and are more sleepy than usual and when awake are irritable. Sunsetting of the eyes and a bulging fontanelle are signs of raised intracranial pressure (ICP). A bruit may be heard over the fontanelle in healthy infants. When there is raised ICP, the skull may act like a blood pressure cuff, producing a bruit. Cerebral bloodflow may also be assessed by Doppler ultrasound. As the ICP rises there is a greater reduction in diastolic than systolic bloodflow. With critically high ICP, there may be a complete cessation of forward and finally a reversal of diastolic bloodflow.

69. **Viral meningitis or encephalitis is a recognised complication of the following viral infections:**
    A. measles.
    B. cytomegalovirus.
    C. Herpes simplex type 1.
    D. Varicella-zoster.
    E. mumps.

70. **Risk factors for development of a brain abscess include:**
    A. pulmonary valve stenosis.
    B. bronchiectasis.
    C. chronic sinusitis.
    D. cyanotic heart disease.
    E. Crohn's disease.

71. **Torticollis is associated with:**
    A. cervical lymphadenitis.
    B. spina bifida occulta.
    C. brainstem tumour.
    D. basal ganglia disease.
    E. intrapartum shoulder dystocia.

72. **In tuberose sclerosis:**
    A. the majority will have multiple pigmented skin lesions.
    B. one of the parents of an affected child will necessarily be affected.
    C. angiofibromas develop on the cheeks during childhood.
    D. all affected children will have severe learning disability.
    E. polycystic kidney disease is a recognised complication.

**69. All of these**

Measles may cause a direct infection of the brain during the acute illness or a later (10–14 days) demyelinating illness, suggesting an immune process. There is commonly a CSF lymphocytosis in mumps and encephalitis, and rarely seizures may be seen 7–10 days into the illness. Herpes simplex type 1 encephalitis is characterised by fever, altered level of consciousness and recurrent fits, which may be focal. Chickenpox may be associated with encephalitis or cerebellaritis presenting as ataxia. Cytomegalovirus may occur as a disseminated infection in neonates and immunocompromised children.

**70. BCD**

Abnormal pulmonary valve leaflets rarely become infected and would embolise to the lungs if this did occur. Infected emboli from chronic pulmonary suppuration may be carried to the brain. In cyanotic heart disease, where septic emboli may be carried through a right to left shunt, there is a recognised risk of cerebral embolus. In chronic sinusitis and chronic otitis there may be direct spread of infection with development of a cerebral abscess. Crohn's disease is not a cause of CNS infection.

**71. ACDE**

A head tilt may provide some relief of pain when cervical lymph nodes are inflamed. A brainstem tumour is a recognised cause of torticollis. Basal ganglia disease may produce bizarre posturing and torticollis may occur. Difficult delivery may cause bleeding into the sternomastoid muscle and later formation of a fibrotic sternomastoid tumour which will cause shortening of the muscle and torticollis.

**72. CE**

Tuberose sclerosis is an autosomal dominant condition which has a high rate of new mutation formation. Parents may therefore be unaffected. Affected children will typically (80%) develop depigmented 'ash leaf' macules over the trunk and limbs – only 20% will develop pigmented lesions. A nodular rash over the nose and cheeks is due to angiofibromas. There is a wide range of intellectual ability in this condition, with some relatively unaffected. Polycystic kidney disease and cardiac rhabdomyomas are also recognised complications. Intracranial calcification in the periventricular region is typical. Fits may occur.

73. **In neurofibromatosis type 1:**
    A. café au lait patches are present from birth.
    B. autosomal recessive inheritance is typical.
    C. the presence of more than seven café au lait patches is diagnostic.
    D. iris hamartomas are present in the majority of affected adolescents.
    E. the risk of CNS tumours is not increased.

74. **Recognised complications of neurofibromatosis type 1 include:**
    A. hypertension.
    B. pathological fractures.
    C. infertility in males.
    D. chronic sinusitis.
    E. paraplegia.

75. **Physical symptoms and signs associated with a myopathy include:**
    A. paraesthesia.
    B. predominantly distal muscle weakness early in the disease.
    C. disturbed bladder function.
    D. muscle fasciculation.
    E. absent reflexes.

76. **Duchenne muscular dystrophy:**
    A. is an inevitably progressive disease.
    B. has an X-linked dominant form of inheritance.
    C. is usually passed from father to son.
    D. presents clinically in new cases between 5 and 10 years of age.
    E. affected patients will be wheelchair-bound by early adolescence.

**73. D**

The café au lait patches characteristic of neurofibromatosis type 1 (NF1) develop during childhood, becoming more obvious by puberty as may the other features – i.e. axillary freckling, iris Lisch nodules (small iris hamartomas) and cutaneous neurofibromas. More than six café au lait patches of greater than 1 cm diameter are diagnostic *when combined* with either one of the other clinical manifestations or a family history. This is an autosomal dominant condition with a high new mutation rate. There is an increased risk of optic nerve gliomas and meningiomas, although CNS tumours are much commoner in NF type 2.

**74. ABE**

Renal artery stenosis and phaeochromocytoma, both associated with hypertension, are recognised complications of NF1. Skeletal abnormality is common in NF, including pathological fractures caused by weakening of the bone by neurofibromas. Neurofibromas occurring within the spinal canal may cause cord compression. Chronic sinusitis and infertility are not features of NF.

**75. None of these**

Myopathies have a history of gradual onset. Standing up and climbing stairs are difficult due to (predominantly) proximal muscle weakness. There is no sensory disturbance, and bladder and bowel function is not affected. Muscle fasciculation is a feature of anterior horn cell and lower motor neuron degeneration, not of myopathy. Absence of reflexes is not a feature of myopathies.

**76. AE**

Duchenne muscular dystrophy (DMD) is an X-linked recessive condition. Only males are affected. There is onset of muscle weakness in infancy. First attempts at walking are delayed and the gait is often clumsy. There is progression of muscle weakness and most boys will be wheelchair-bound by the early teenage years. Young men with DMD usually die before reproduction is possible. Theoretically males can only pass on their affected X chromosome to their daughters (all carriers), whereas females can pass on their X chromosomes to either their daughters (50% carriers) or to their sons (50% affected).

77. **The following results would be direct evidence of an underlying muscle disorder:**
   A. low plasma calcium level.
   B. elevated CSF protein level.
   C. fibrillation potentials on EMG.
   D. raised plasma ammonia.
   E. elevated plasma creatinine.

78. **Indications for early back surgery to close the defect in a newborn with spina bifida cystica include:**
   A. a bulging fontanelle.
   B. voluntary movement of the legs.
   C. patulous anus.
   D. crying on painful stimulus to the foot.
   E. rupture of the meningeal sac.

79. **Long-term complications of bacterial meningitis include:**
   A. mental retardation.
   B. 'petit mal' epilepsy.
   C. deafness.
   D. communicating hydrocephalus.
   E. paraplegia.

80. **In Guillain–Barré syndrome the following clinical signs and symptoms are recognised:**
   A. facial palsy.
   B. hypertension.
   C. diplopia.
   D. muscle and back pains.
   E. difficulty swallowing secretions.

**77. None of these**

There are few tests which will give direct evidence of a myopathy. Diagnosis is usually based on the history, family history, clinical features and muscle biopsy findings. Plasma creatine phosphokinase levels are raised in Duchenne muscular dystrophy. Hypocalcaemia may cause muscle weakness or predispose to muscle spasm or tetany. An elevated CSF protein level is suggestive of CNS inflammation rather than primary muscle disease. Fibrillation potentials are the EMG manifestation of muscle fasciculation caused by denervation and are not due to primary muscle disease. Abnormalities of plasma ammonia and creatinine are not characteristic of muscle disease.

**78. BD**

The main reason for early surgery in spina bifida is to preserve cord function. If there is voluntary leg movement or preservation of sensation, then early surgery is indicated. An open back lesion with good nursing care will not necessarily become infected, but closure will reduce the risk of infection. A bulging fontanelle may indicate a significant degree of hydrocephalus. A patulous anus suggests that there is extensive damage to the lower cord. Surgeons will not be keen to shunt hydrocephalus until an open back lesion has been closed and the risk of meningitis reduced. Infected shunts have to be removed and replaced after treatment.

**79. ACD**

Mental retardation (uncommon), deafness (3%) and hydrocephalus are all recognised late complications of bacterial meningitis. 'Petit mal' epilepsy is a genetic epilepsy and would not be expected after meningitis. Paraplegia would be an exceptionally rare complication.

**80. ABCDE**

Sensory loss is uncommon in Guillain–Barré syndrome. Bulbar palsy and weakness of the extraocular muscles of the eye may occur in more severe cases. Muscle and back pains are quite common. Hypertension may occur if the autonomic nervous system is affected.

81. **The following signs and symptoms would be present in a 3-year-old with severe lead poisoning:**
    A. anaemia.
    B. lead lines on the gums.
    C. papilloedema.
    D. a history of abdominal pain or constipation.
    E. swelling and tenderness at the ends of the long bones and ribs.

82. **The following antibiotics will effectively cross the blood/brain barrier and can be given intravenously to treat bacterial meningitis:**
    A. benzyl penicillin.
    B. gentamicin.
    C. cefotaxime.
    D. chloramphenicol.
    E. vancomycin.

**81. ACD**
Lead poisoning is associated with anaemia, abdominal pain and constipation. Headaches and vomiting are symptoms of incipient encephalopathy and raised intracranial pressure (ICP). Lead lines on the gums occur in adults where there is associated gum disease (producing lead sulphides) but not in children. Swelling of the ends of the long bones is a feature of rickets. In lead poisoning there is deposition of lead at the ends of the long bones which shows on X-ray.

**82. ACD**
Penicillin crosses the inflamed blood/brain barrier well and is the first-choice antibiotic for Pneumococcal and Meningococcal meningitis. Chloramphenicol and cefotaxime cross the blood/brain barrier well and are used for Haemophilus and gram-negative meningitis. Chloramphenicol is not a first-choice antibiotic. Aminoglycosides and vancomycin do not cross the blood/brain barrier well, but special intrathecal preparations may be used if there is access to the CSF.

# 5

## Urogenital

1. **Daytime wetting (lack of bladder control):**
   A. is considered normal in children of less than 3 years of age.
   B. occurs in less than 5% of 5-year-olds.
   C. is caused by organic disease in more than 90% of children who had previously achieved bladder control.
   D. can be associated with giggling.
   E. due to a non-organic behavioural cause; it is commoner in boys than girls.

2. **Renal scarring due to urinary tract infection:**
   A. is commoner in girls than boys.
   B. is more likely to develop in children under 2 years of age than in children over 6 years.
   C. is prevented by long-term prophylactic antibiotics.
   D. affects the left kidney more commonly than the right.
   E. occurs only if symptoms of urine infection are neglected.

3. **Vesico-ureteric reflux can reliably be detected by:**
   A. careful clinical examination.
   B. DMSA isotope scan.
   C. ultrasound scan.
   D. micturating cystourethrogram (MCUG).
   E. intravenous pyelogram (IVP).

4. **Urinary tract infection (after the neonatal period):**
   A. is caused by haematogenous spread of infection to the kidneys.
   B. is diagnosed by finding $> 10^5$ white blood cells/ml urine.
   C. occurs more commonly in girls than boys.
   D. is caused by enterococci in $> 50\%$ cases.
   E. can be diagnosed only by suprapubic bladder aspiration in children under 2 years.

1. **ABDE**
   Most (>75%) children will achieve daytime bladder control by the age of 3 years. More than 95% of children will be dry by day by 4 years. Girls are likely to be toilet-trained earlier than boys. Reflux of urine into the vagina and giggle incontinence may also cause daytime wetting. Organic pathology accounts for only 5% of diurnal enuresis. Secondary enuresis is most likely to be due to emotional factors, but is more likely than primary enuresis to be due to organic pathology.

2. **ABC**
   Renal scarring is caused when infected urine refluxes into the kidney (*intrarenal* reflux) causing a pyelonephritis. Once detected, renal scarring does not usually progress significantly. This suggests either that the immature kidney is more susceptible to damage or that urine infections are more easily diagnosed and treated in older children. Neither kidney has increased susceptibility to scarring.

3. **DE**
   Reflux cannot be detected by clinical examination. DMSA isotope is taken up by functioning renal tubules and so demonstrates renal scarring (cold spots) but not reflux. Ultrasound scanning will usually miss mild or moderate reflux and will show reflux only if it is severe or if reflux occurs during scanning. A micturating cystourethrogram is the best method for assessing reflux before voluntary bladder control has been achieved. MAG3 and DTPA isotope scans will demonstrate urinary drainage and the presence of reflux in older children. An IVP may show reflux but higher doses of radiation are involved and there is a risk of reaction to the contrast.

4. **C**
   Urinary tract infections (UTI) arise from ascending infections. The organisms causing UTI are bowel organisms, predominantly *E. coli*. Although white blood cells (WBC) are usually present in infected urine, a pure growth of organisms $>10^5$/ml in a midstream urine sample is required to diagnose a UTI. Urine infection is commoner in girls than boys outside the neonatal period. Urine samples in young children, obtained by applying an adherent bag to the perineum, should ideally be repeated or a suprapubic sample obtained before diagnosing a UTI. Positive clean catch urine samples should be regarded as accurate.

5. **In 'uncomplicated' acute pyelonephritis:**
   A. the ability of the kidneys to concentrate the urine is reduced.
   B. the plasma creatinine level will increase to more than double.
   C. the kidneys will appear echogenic on ultrasound scan.
   D. the patient is invariably febrile.
   E. renal sodium losses are increased.

6. **Predisposing factors for the development of urine infections include:**
   A. bladder diverticulum.
   B. posterior urethral valves.
   C. phimosis.
   D. vesico-ureteric reflux.
   E. giggle incontinence.

7. **A 5-year-old girl has been shown to have mild vesico-ureteric reflux, no renal scarring and recurrent urinary tract infections. Appropriate management would be:**
   A. referral for surgical reimplantation of the ureters.
   B. intermittent courses of antibiotics for treatment of symptomatic infection.
   C. long-term trimethoprim at bedtime.
   D. referral for endoscopic 'STING' operation.
   E. discharge from follow-up.

8. **In acute renal failure the following tests are of value in diagnosing the underlying cause:**
   A. stool culture.
   B. blood film and coagulation screen.
   C. urine microscopy.
   D. plasma creatinine level.
   E. renal ultrasound scan.

5. **ACE**

Symptoms do not permit doctors reliably to distinguish pyelonephritis from cystitis. Patients with recurrent pyelonephritis may become 'tolerant' of infection with time, and fever may not always be a feature. In acute pyelonephritis renal tubular function will be affected and renal concentrating power and ability to retain sodium will be diminished. Unless there is severe renal damage, creatinine concentration will not be significantly affected. Kidneys will appear bright on ultrasound scan.

6. **ABD**

Any anatomical abnormality causing failure of complete drainage of the urinary system results in an increased risk of urine infection. Phimosis does not result in failure of bladder emptying and so does not increase the risk of urine infection. Phimosis may be associated with dysuria caused by local infection. Giggle incontinence may cause perineal irritation, but should not increase the risk of UTI.

7. **BCD**

Children with severe reflux causing dilatation and tortuosity of the ureter and clubbing of the calyces should be referred for surgical treatment. First-choice surgical treatment would be a STING procedure, with submucosal, paraureteric injection of silicone. If the STING procedure failed, then ureteric reimplantation may be appropriate. Milder grades of reflux usually improve spontaneously. In this child the risk of scarring is small and either intermittent treatment of infections or long-term antibiotics may be appropriate. Discharge from follow-up would be inappropriate as further assessment will be necessary.

8. **ABCE**

Investigations in acute renal failure should determine any reversible factors. Stool culture may demonstrate a verocytotoxin producing *E. coli* 018, which may trigger the haemolytic uraemic syndrome (HUS). A blood film will show haemolysis and give a platelet count. Thrombocytopenia is usual in HUS but the coagulation screen is usually normal – both are abnormal in conditions causing DIC. A pyelonephritis may precipitate renal failure, especially if renal function is already compromised. A renal ultrasound scan will exclude any obstruction of the urinary tract. Plasma creatinine will document poor renal function without giving clues as to its cause.

9. **Hyperkalaemia requires treatment if the ECG shows:**
   A. inversion of T-waves in the right ventricular leads.
   B. multifocal ventricular ectopic beats.
   C. left ventricular hypertrophy.
   D. widened QRS complex.
   E. a short PR interval.

10. **Recognised treatment of hyperkalaemia causing ECG changes include intravenous administration of:**
   A. phosphate.
   B. calcium.
   C. salbutamol.
   D. calcium resonium.
   E. sodium bicarbonate.

11. **Conditions associated with an elevated anion gap include:**
   A. ingestion of antifreeze.
   B. diabetic ketoacidosis.
   C. chronic respiratory failure.
   D. chronic renal failure.
   E. shock.

12. **Consequences of heavy proteinuria in the nephrotic syndrome include:**
   A. hypertension.
   B. oedema.
   C. tendency to thrombosis.
   D. increased risk of infection.
   E. cardiac failure.

9. **BD**

The ECG in hyperkalaemia progresses from tall peaked T-waves to broadening of the QRS complex with extrasystoles and arrhythmias to bradycardia, hypotension and cardiac arrest. Oliguria itself does not inevitably indicate the presence of hyperkalaemia.

10. **BCE**

Suspected hyperkalaemia is one of the real indications for the use of calcium in the treatment of cardiac arrest. Intravenous calcium reduces myocardial irritability in hyperkalaemia. Intravenous salbutamol will cause temporary lowering of plasma potassium. Calcium resonium is an ion exchange resin which binds potassium but cannot be administered intravenously; it is usually given into the GI tract – i.e. stomach and/or rectum. In situations where there is a metabolic acidosis, potassium leaks out of the cells. Correction of the acidosis with bicarbonate will produce a lowering of potassium levels. Insulin and dextrose given intravenously will also lower potassium levels. If the cause is not immediately reversible, all of the above measures are useful in the short term only, until some form of dialysis can be instituted.

11. **ABDE**

The anion gap is the difference between the concentration of major anions and cations. In practice, the anion gap = $Na^+ - (Cl^- + HCO_3^-)$. The normal anion gap is $< 10\,mmol/L$. An increased anion gap is found when there is an excess of organic acids (as in some inborn errors of metabolism – e.g. glutaric acid, propionic acid), lactic acid (shock), ketoacids (starvation and diabetes), renal failure or where there is an excess of exogenous acids as in some poisonings – e.g. aspirin, methanol and ethylene glycol.

12. **BCD**

Hypertension is unusual in nephrotic syndrome in children and is not due to the hypoproteinaemia, but to the underlying renal lesion. Oedema is directly related to the low plasma oncotic pressure. An increased tendency to thrombosis may result from hyperviscosity combined with elevated levels of fibrinogen and lowered levels of fibrinolytic factors such as antithrombin III. Susceptibility to infection with Pneumococci results from loss of immunoglobulin and the effects of high-dose steroids, which may reduce resistance to and mask early signs of infection.

13. **Infections associated with nephritis include:**
    A. hepatitis B.
    B. mumps.
    C. group B Streptococci.
    D. malaria.
    E. Pneumococcal pneumonia.

14. **A 4-year-old boy has a history of polyuria for 1 year and a normal physical examination. First-line investigation should include:**
    A. water-deprivation test.
    B. urinalysis.
    C. 24-hour urine collection for estimation of creatinine clearance.
    D. glucose tolerance test.
    E. morning urine sample for osmolarity.

15. **Features of Henoch-Schönlein purpura include:**
    A. thrombocytopenia.
    B. increased susceptibility to infection.
    C. arthritis affecting large joints.
    D. blood in the stools.
    E. intracranial haemorrhage.

16. **Renal enlargement is associated with:**
    A. tuberose sclerosis.
    B. cystic fibrosis.
    C. diabetic ketoacidosis.
    D. pyelonephritis.
    E. hemihypertrophy.

13. **AD**

Hepatitis B and malaria are both associated with a membranous nephropathy. Group A beta-haemolytic Streptococci infections are associated with a proliferative glomerulonephritis. Group B Streptococci infections are typically a neonatal problem. Complications of mumps infection include meningitis, encephalitis, deafness, facial palsy, orchitis, pancreatitis, myocarditis, hepatitis, thyroiditis, ITP and sternal oedema, but not usually a nephritis. Pneumococcal infections are occasionally associated with the haemolytic uraemic syndrome, but not nephritis.

14. **BE**

One could argue that this child should have no investigations at all. The commonest cause for excessive thirst is habit. Young children with habitual polydipsia often sleep through the night without drinks. Children with an inability to concentrate their urine are compulsory drinkers and cannot last overnight without drinks. Initial investigations for this child should include urinalysis, urine culture and a morning urine sample for osmolarity. If the child is unable to produce a concentrated morning urine sample of > 600 mosm/kg (without any enforced fluid restriction), then a urine concentrating problem is more likely. Check plasma electrolytes, calcium and creatinine levels and carry out a formal water-deprivation test.

15. **CD**

The purpuric rash of Henoch-Schönlein purpura is caused by a vasculitis, not by reduced platelet numbers or function. There is a flitting arthritis, with pain and swelling affecting predominantly the large joints. There may be severe colicky abdominal pain as the vasculitis may affect the bowel wall. There may be rectal bleeding, and occasionally colicky pain results from the development of an intussusception. Involvement of the CNS is a very rare feature of the disease, usually without intracranial haemorrhage.

16. **ADE**

Tuberose sclerosis is associated with renal polycystic disease. Pyelonephritis is associated with acute swelling and 'bright' – echogenic kidneys on ultrasound. Hemihypertrophy is associated with an increased risk of Wilms tumour (nephroblastoma) in preschool children.

17. **Proteinuria is associated with:**
    A. fever.
    B. diabetes insipidus.
    C. urinary tract infection.
    D. exercise.
    E. hypokalaemia.

18. **A 4-month-old boy requires surgery if he is found to have:**
    A. a non-retractile foreskin.
    B. bilateral hydroceles.
    C. a left inguinal hernia.
    D. an undescended right testis.
    E. an umbilical hernia.

19. **A child receiving long-term steroid therapy for nephrotic syndrome is at increased risk of:**
    A. cataract.
    B. hypertension.
    C. Varicella-zoster infection.
    D. avascular necrosis of the hip.
    E. hirsutism.

20. **A 6-year-old child presents with a history of bloody diarrhoea and vomiting 10 days before presentation to hospital. After 6 days, the symptoms settled, but 3 days later the vomiting recurred associated with troublesome nosebleeds. The child appeared pale and slightly jaundiced, but was not pyrexial. Likely findings on investigation will include:**
    A. disseminated intravascular coagulation.
    B. raised creatinine level.
    C. raised liver enzyme levels.
    D. low platelet count.
    E. red cell fragments on blood film.

**17. ACD**

Proteinuria is significant at more than $4-6\,mg/m^2/hour$ – i.e. $>150\,mg$ protein/day. In the nephrotic syndrome protein excretion exceeds $40\,mg/m^2/hour$. Exercise and fever may cause increased urinary protein loss. In orthostatic proteinuria protein losses are increased in the upright position, but a urine sample collected on wakening should be protein-free. Urinary tract infection with accompanying inflammation will usually be associated with proteinuria.

**18. C**

A non-retractile foreskin is a normal finding in preschool boys. Hydroceles and umbilical hernias of varying sizes are a common finding in routine baby checks in the first few months of life. These rarely persist and do not require treatment unless persisting beyond the 1st year. Inguinal hernias should always be referred for surgery because of the risk of incarceration. Undescended testes are common, but should be referred if still not fully descended by 1 year, as ultrastructural changes may occur in the seminiferous tubules of the undescended testis during the 2nd year.

**19. ABCDE – all of these**

These are well-recognised complications of long-term oral steroid therapy. Children on oral steroid should carry a steroid card, and should be given extra steroid if exposed to 'stress' as in severe infection or serious accident. A child on oral steroids, who is not known to have protective antibody levels and who has been personally in contact with another child with chickenpox, should be given Zoster hyperimmune gammaglobulin (ZIG) by IM injection as soon as possible and certainly within 48 hours. Acyclovir should be given if chickenpox develops.

**20. BDE**

This is a classic story for a child with the haemolytic uraemic syndrome. *E. coli* 018 may produce a verocytotoxin, which is toxic to vascular endothelium. Disruption of the micro-circulation occurs and platelet consumption and red cell fragmentation result. Haemolysis, jaundice, anaemia and thrombocytopenia occur with later development of oliguria and renal failure.

# 6

## Metabolic

1. **Phenylketonuria (PKU):**
   A. is detected by raised phenylalanine levels on the Guthrie test.
   B. should be treated with a phenylalanine-free diet.
   C. classically causes pale irises and fair skin.
   D. results in IQ loss of 40–60 points by 1 year of age in the untreated child.
   E. causes females to be infertile.

2. **An inborn error of metabolism should be considered in a sick baby:**
   A. if the blood urea level is less than 1 mmol/L.
   B. with a metabolic acidosis.
   C. if the parents are consanguineous.
   D. who is hypoglycaemic in the neonatal period.
   E. with hepatosplenomegaly.

3. **A child with severe albinism (tyrosinase-negative):**
   A. will have no pigmented naevi.
   B. will have red irises.
   C. will never develop significant skin pigmentation.
   D. will have nystagmus and photophobia.
   E. should avoid sunlight.

4. **A high blood ammonia level:**
   A. gives a patient a typical ammoniacal smell.
   B. occurs with urea cycle defects.
   C. is present in Reye syndrome.
   D. presents with coma and acute metabolic crisis.
   E. is reduced by a high-protein diet.

1. **ACD**

   PKU is detected by finding an elevated level of phenylalanine on dried blood spots (Guthrie cards) collected from all babies at the end of the 1st week of life. The incidence is 1 in 10 000–20 000 Caucasian births. The treatment is by limiting the oral intake of phenylalanine. The outcome for the untreated child is microcephaly, convulsions and cerebral atrophy, with a significant loss in IQ even by 1 year of age. Women with PKU can conceive but must adhere to a low-phenylalanine diet as during pregnancy, even mildly elevated phenylalanine levels result in fetal damage.

2. **ABCDE**

   Inborn errors of metabolism (IEM) are rare, but should be considered in any sick child. There is an increased incidence in consanguineous marriages due to autosomal recessive inheritance. Metabolic acidosis may be due to accumulation of organic acids. A low blood urea level or high ammonia level may indicate a defect in the urea cycle. Persistent hypoglycaemia in the neonatal period may be due to an inborn error of metabolism. Hepatosplenomegaly may result from a storage defect.

3. **ACDE**

   In children with severe (tyrosinase-negative) albinism the absence of pigment (melanin) is complete and permanent. They have very pale hair and skin, no pigmented naevi or freckles and there is an increased risk of skin neoplasia. The iris is always blue or grey. There is nystagmus and photophobia, and most patients are legally blind. Lack of iris pigment produces a red pupillary reflex. Sunlight should be avoided, both for comfort and to reduce the risk of skin neoplasia.

4. **BCD**

   An average diet contains excess of nitrogen (from protein), which is mainly excreted as urea. Enzymatic defects of all steps of the urea cycle have been described resulting in high blood ammonia. High ammonia levels are toxic to the brain, resulting in rapid neurological deterioration, apnoea and coma. High protein diets exacerbate the problem. In Reye syndrome liver mitochondrial damage disrupts the urea cycle. The patients do not smell of ammonia.

5. **Reye syndrome:**
   A. presents with acute encephalopathy and raised intracranial pressure.
   B. typically occurs after a mild viral infection.
   C. results from a self-limiting abnormality of mitochondrial function.
   D. may be ameliorated by aspirin therapy.
   E. has a mortality rate of 40%.

6. **A sick baby is suspected of having galactosaemia because of the following:**
   A. collapse with *E. coli* sepsis.
   B. metabolic acidosis prior to milk ingestion.
   C. cataracts.
   D. the urine is positive for reducing sugars.
   E. elevated serum lactose level.

7. **The following biochemical abnormalities should alert the physician to the following diagnoses:**
   A. high conjugated hyperbilirubinaemia is typical of Crigler–Najjar syndrome.
   B. high serum ferritin indicates iron deficiency anaemia.
   C. low serum sodium and Addison's disease.
   D. glucose-6-phosphate dehydrogenase deficiency manifests as acute haemolytic crises.
   E. low serum zinc and acrodermatitis enteropathica.

8. **The following clinical features occur in the glycogen storage disease:**
   A. hepatosplenomegaly.
   B. fasting hypoglycaemia.
   C. myopathy.
   D. mental retardation.
   E. lactic acidosis.

5. **ABCE**

Reye syndrome is a rare, acute, frequently fatal encephalopathy of unknown cause occurring in children of any age. There is an abnormality of hepatic mitochondrial function lasting 2–6 days. Reye syndrome presents with encephalopathy and liver dysfunction – e.g. raised serum transaminases, hypoglycaemia, prolonged prothrombin time or raised ammonia. A range of inborn errors of metabolism may present in a similar manner. The illness typically occurs after a mild viral illness. Other factors, such as aspirin, have also been implicated in the pathogenesis.

6. **ACD**

A baby with galactosaemia will become ill following the introduction of lactose in milk which is the main source of dietary galactose. The enzyme defect causes elevated levels of galactose-1-phosphate which is toxic to the liver, kidney, lens and brain. The symptoms mimic severe sepsis but babies are also at increased risk of severe infection – e.g. *E. coli* septicaemia. The urine is positive for reducing substances (galactose), detectable by clinitest. The treatment is total elimination of galactose and lactose from the diet.

7. **CDE**

An unconjugated hyperbilirubinaemia is seen in Crigler–Najjar syndrome due to absence of glucuronyl transferase and an inability to conjugate bilirubin. Iron deficiency anaemia is typified by low serum ferritin. Lack of mineralocorticoids in Addison's disease causes hyponatraemia. G6PD deficiency results in acute haemolytic crises that are triggered by a variety of oxidant factors. Low serum zinc causes a typical exudative skin rash on the face and napkin area – acrodermatitis enteropathica.

8. **ABCE**

Enzyme defects in the glycogen degradation pathway may raise the glycogen content of the organ in which the enzyme is localised, mainly the liver or muscle. Enzyme defects in the liver are usually characterised by hypoglycaemia, whereas the muscle defects are characterised by myopathy. Cerebral function is usually normal so long as hypoglycaemic damage is prevented. The degradation of glycogen to pyruvate is intact and therefore chronic lactic acidaemia is usual.

**9. For children with mucopolysaccharidosis:**

   **A.** the course of the disease is typified by acute exacerbations with periods of remission.

   **B.** the clinical features are present at birth.

   **C.** recurrent respiratory infections occur.

   **D.** congestive heart failure results from congenital heart disease.

   **E.** the presentation may be with claw hand deformity.

**9.  CE**

The mucopolysaccharidoses are one group of many lysosomal storage disorders. Lysosomes contain acid hydrolases which degrade a variety of macromolecules. Defective function of any of these hydrolases results in intra-lysosomal accumulation of the unhydrolysed substrates, in this case mucopolysaccharides. The phenotype is very variable, but is characterised by a progressive course due to increasing accumulation of the macromolecules in the tissues causing multisystem involvement. Accumulation in the tissues of the upper airway results in increasing obstruction and respiratory failure. Accumulation in the myocardium and valves results in heart failure. For some children with milder forms the initial presentation may be with claw hand deformity.

# 7

# Hepatology

1. **Important liver functions include:**
   A. maintenance of blood glucose concentration.
   B. control of insulin release.
   C. excretion of nitrogen waste as ammonia.
   D. production of gammaglobulin.
   E. 25 hydroxylation of vitamin D.

2. **A 6-year-old girl presents with acute infectious hepatitis. Over the course of several days, she develops increasing jaundice and becomes confused and at times aggressive. At first, the liver is enlarged, and then decreases in size:**
   A. there will be a predominantly unconjugated hyperbilirubin-aemia.
   B. the patient is at risk of hypoglycaemia.
   C. reduction of the size of the liver, in this case, indicates early improvement in the child's condition.
   D. the bleeding time will be prolonged.
   E. a haematemesis will worsen any encephalopathy.

3. **A 3-week-old breast-fed baby presents with increasing jaundice and failure to thrive. The stools are light coloured and the urine is dark in colour:**
   A. the most likely diagnosis is breast milk jaundice.
   B. a liver ultrasound scan will exclude biliary atresia.
   C. tenfold elevation in ALT (SGOT) indicates a neonatal hepatitis.
   D. excretion of HIDA (or DISIDA) isotope into the duodenum excludes biliary atresia.
   E. a liver biopsy is required if the isotope scan shows no excretion of isotope into the bowel.

4. **The following would be compatible with a diagnosis of portal hypertension:**
   A. history of use of neonatal umbilical venous catheters.
   B. thrombocytosis.
   C. haematemesis.
   D. iron deficiency anaemia.
   E. prolonged prothrombin time.

1. **AE**

   Liver functions include synthesis, detoxification, excretion and metabolic regulation. Regulation of glucose homeostasis includes glycogenolysis and glyconeogenesis. Cholecalciferol is 25 hydroxylated by the liver before further hydroxylation by the kidneys. Insulin release is regulated by the pancreas. Gamma-globulins are produced by plasma cells throughout the body. Nitrogenous waste is excreted by the liver but as urea rather than as ammonia.

2. **BE**

   The clinical picture is of evolving liver failure, and a worsening clinical picture. There is a high risk of hypoglycaemia. Liver swelling results in an obstructive jaundice with failure of excretion of conjugated bilirubin. A coagulation profile will show prolongation of the prothrombin and partial thromboplastin time. The bleeding time will be normal so long as platelet numbers and function are preserved. A haematemesis introduces a large protein load into the bowel, increasing levels of ammonia and worsening the encephalopathy.

3. **DE**

   Either biliary atresia or neonatal hepatitis are the most likely diagnoses. Neither liver ultrasound scan nor liver enzymes reliably distinguish between the two conditions. An isotope scan performed after phenobarbitone induction of liver enzymes will exclude biliary atresia if there is excretion of isotope into the bowel. If no isotope is excreted, a liver biopsy will confirm the diagnosis of biliary atresia. If the diagnosis is confirmed, a Kasai hepatic porto-enterostomy will be performed in an attempt to re-establish bile flow.

4. **ACD**

   Neonatal umbilical venous catheters may introduce infection and increase the risk of thrombosis in the upper portal vein, leading to a risk of portal hypertension. Increased portal venous pressure will result in the development of varices with the consequent risk of haematemesis. Persistent bleeding from varices may result in iron deficiency anaemia. Splenomegaly is associated with hypersplenism and thrombocytopenia as platelets become sequestered within the spleen. So long as liver cell synthetic function is preserved, the prothrombin time will be normal.

5. **Investigation of conjugated neonatal hyperbilirubinaemia should include:**
   A. jejunal biopsy.
   B. endoscopic retrograde cholangiography.
   C. plain abdominal X-ray.
   D. testing for cystic fibrosis.
   E. isotope liver scan.

6. **Hepatomegaly is a feature of:**
   A. coeliac disease.
   B. bronchiolitis.
   C. hydatid abscess.
   D. beta-thalassaemia.
   E. type 1 glycogen storage disease.

7. **Pancreatitis:**
   A. is characterised by an increased plasma amylase level.
   B. may follow blunt abdominal trauma.
   C. is associated with hypercalcaemia.
   D. is a recognised complication of mumps infection.
   E. is a recognised complication of cystic fibrosis.

8. **Calcification seen on plain abdominal X-ray is associated with:**
   A. neuroblastoma.
   B. ingestion of iron tablets.
   C. dermoid tumour of the liver.
   D. appendicitis.
   E. renal stones.

**5. DE**

Jejunal biopsy has no role in the investigation of neonatal hyperbilirubinaemia. ERCP is not practical in neonates. Plain abdominal X-ray is unlikely to be helpful. Liver imaging by ultrasound and radioisotope are the modalities of choice. Diagnostic testing in this clinical situation is directed to excluding infections, metabolic abnormality, endocrine disorder, bile duct obstruction and other conditions – e.g. cystic fibrosis. Sweat testing is not usually reliable within the neonatal period; CF testing should be by alternative means such as gene testing.

**6. CDE**

Hepatomegaly is not a feature of coeliac disease. In bronchiolitis the liver is often displaced downwards by hyperinflated lungs, but it is not enlarged. In thalassaemia the chronic anaemia results in extramedullary haematopoiesis causing enlargement of the liver and spleen. Hydatid cysts may cause significant enlargement of the liver. There is significant liver enlargement in most of the glycogen storage diseases except where the enzyme deficiency predominantly affects muscle.

**7. ABCDE**

Pancreatitis is diagnosed when there is abdominal pain sometimes radiating through to the back, abdominal tenderness, vomiting, fever and jaundice. The serum amylase is usually raised. A pancreatic cyst or pseudocyst (with a fluid collection in the lesser sac) may develop after an acute episode. Acute pancreatitis may occur in children after viral infection (e.g. mumps) and also in association with biliary disease, cystic fibrosis, abdominal trauma, choledocal cysts, gallstones, hypercalcaemia, malnutrition and drugs. Hypocalcaemia is common.

**8. ACDE**

Iron tablets are radio-opaque but not because of calcification. In young children calcification in the suprarenal region is very suggestive of neuroblastoma. Dermoid tumours wherever they occur are likely to contain calcified material. In acute appendicitis a calcified faecolith may be seen in the region of the appendix. Renal stones are usually associated with infection and will be radio-opaque due to calcium content.

9. **Causes of acute liver failure include:**
   A. white spirit (turps substitute) ingestion.
   B. Addison's disease.
   C. measles infection.
   D. Wilson's disease.
   E. paracetamol ingestion.

10. **The following are complications of acute liver failure:**
    A. hyperkalaemia.
    B. cerebral oedema.
    C. haematemesis.
    D. thrombocytopenia.
    E. hyperglycaemia.

11. **Reye syndrome is associated with:**
    A. fatty infiltration of the liver.
    B. altered level of consciousness.
    C. progressive jaundice.
    D. chickenpox infection.
    E. prior aspirin ingestion.

12. **Causes of conjugated hyperbilirubinaemia include:**
    A. total parenteral nutrition.
    B. prematurity.
    C. glucuronyl transferase deficiency.
    D. infectious hepatitis.
    E. choledochal cyst.

9. **DE**

Turps substitute does not affect the liver as it is not absorbed from the bowel. Liver failure is not a feature of Addison's disease or measles. In Wilson's disease there is a failure of normal copper transport and excessive copper deposition in the tissues. Acute, chronic and acute fulminating hepatitis with liver failure may all occur in Wilson's disease – the latter sometimes as the presenting feature of this autosomal recessive condition. Paracetamol is hepatotoxic in overdose, with acute liver failure developing after 5–6 days.

10. **BC**

In acute liver failure, failure of hepatic glucose metabolism results in a tendency to hypoglycaemia. The stress of the severe illness may cause gastric erosions with a tendency to haematemesis. The failure of liver synthetic activity will exacerbate the coagulopathy. Encephalopathy is a common feature of liver failure. The early signs of encephalopathy and cerebral oedema include vomiting due to raised intracranial pressure. Hypokalaemia is common in liver failure.

11. **ABDE**

In Reye syndrome there is disruption of normal mitochondrial function. This disease has become progressively less common over the past 10 years since the use of aspirin for the management of febrile illness in children has been banned. Reye syndrome has been associated with many virus infections, including chickenpox and influenza. Fatty infiltration of the liver is common. Diagnostic features include elevation of hepatic transaminases, ammonia and abnormal coagulation combined with an encephalopathy. Progressive jaundice is not a feature.

12. **ADE**

Obstructive jaundice may result from sludge in the biliary tree as may occur in babies on long-term parenteral nutrition, liver swelling as in infectious hepatitis or from anatomical obstruction such as with a cyst in the biliary tree or biliary atresia. Unconjugated hyperbilirubinaemia may result from deficiency of hepatic glucuronyl transferase (Crigler–Najjar syndrome) or from transient immaturity of hepatic bilirubin conjugation as in prematurity.

13. **Causes of splenomegaly include:**
    A. EB virus infection.
    B. CMV infection.
    C. portal hypertension.
    D. ventricular septal defect.
    E. congenital spherocytosis.

14. **Hepatitis A:**
    A. is an enterovirus.
    B. is spread by aerosol droplets.
    C. has no chronic carrier state.
    D. can be prevented by passive immunisation with immune globulin.
    E. has an incubation period of 6 weeks.

15. **Hepatitis B:**
    A. is best diagnosed by viral culture.
    B. can be transmitted from mother to baby.
    C. is most infectious if the patient is HBsAg-positive and HbeAg-negative.
    D. may be prevented by active immunisation.
    E. does not cause chronic infection in children.

16. **Gallstones in childhood:**
    A. should be removed once detected.
    B. are best diagnosed by ultrasound scan.
    C. are found in cystic fibrosis.
    D. are found by spherocytosis.
    E. are found in Crohn's disease.

13.  **ABCE**
Splenomegaly is a part of many virus infections. In EBV and
CMV infections splenomegaly and lymphadenopathy are
common. It is very unlikely that a child has portal hypertension
unless there is clear-cut splenomegaly. There is no reason for a
child with an uncomplicated VSD to have splenomegaly unless
there is an intercurrent virus infection or bacterial endocarditis.

14.  **ACD**
Hepatitis A belongs to the picornavirus (RNA) group of
enteroviruses. The virus is spread by the faeco-oral route and
may occur in epidemics in overcrowded conditions. The
infection may be prevented by administration of immune
globulin (where time is limited) or by active immunisation with
inactivated virus. There is an incubation period of up to 4
weeks. There is no chronic carrier state.

15.  **BD**
Transmission of Hepatitis B infection from mother to baby
occurs, probably at the time of delivery rather than by
transplacental spread of infection. Mothers who are core
antigen positive are the most infectious. Babies born to mothers
who are HBsAg positive should be immunised with intramuscular immunoglobulin within 24 hours of delivery, and should
start a programme of active immunisation. Children may
become chronic carriers in just the same way as in adults. The
chronic carrier state is more likely to develop in children who
are malnourished, immunosuppressed or immunodeficient.
Positive serology tests indicate exposure to the virus – infectivity,
chronic carriage or immunity is then assessed by more detailed
study of the pattern of antigen and antibody serology results.

16.  **BCDE**
Gallstones are uncommon in children. Stones may occur where
there is biliary sludging as in cystic fibrosis or biliary infection.
Pigment stones are likely to occur where there is ongoing
haemolysis. Ultrasonography (USS) is the best imaging method.
Stones whether radiolucent or not will be detected easily by
USS; stones will cast an ultrasound 'shadow' which will be seen
on the scan. Most gallstones are asymptomatic and therefore
require no treatment.

# 8

# Orthopaedics and rheumatology

1. **In newborn infants:**
   A. postural talipes equinovarus can be expected to correct spontaneously without treatment.
   B. fixed talipes equinovarus requires surgical treatment in the majority of cases.
   C. screening for congenital dislocation of the hips is performed by obtaining a plain radiograph of the pelvis.
   D. congenital dislocation of the hips is more common in those delivered in a breech presentation.
   E. physiological lumbar lordosis is present.

2. **In diagnosis and treatment of congenital dislocation of the hips (CDH):**
   A. the Ortolani test involves flexion of the hips and knees to 90° followed by abduction of the hips.
   B. limitation of full abduction of one hip in a 1-year-old child who has an abnormal gait would suggest a diagnosis of CDH.
   C. ultrasound examination of the hips can be used to diagnose CDH.
   D. early detection and splinting will produce a good result in most cases.
   E. delay in the diagnosis and treatment until after the child has begun to walk will result in a higher incidence of permanent joint abnormality.

3. **The following are benign postural variants:**
   A. sternomastoid torticollis in a 3-year-old.
   B. bow legs with tibial torsion in a 2-year-old.
   C. knock knees in a 5-year-old.
   D. out-toeing in an 11-month-old.
   E. a thoracic scoliosis of 40° in a 13-year-old boy.

4. **The following are risk factors for the development of scoliosis:**
   A. male sex in adolescence.
   B. Marfan syndrome.
   C. muscular dystrophy.
   D. spina bifida.
   E. cerebral palsy.

1. **ABD**

   Talipes equinovarus is a common postural variant in the newborn consisting of plantar flexion at the ankle and inversion of the foot. If the deformity cannot be corrected passively, then the talipes is fixed and requires treatment. Splints and serial plastering may be helpful but the majority of patients require surgery. The spine of the normal newborn infant forms a single curve (convex posteriorly) and the physiological cervical and lumbar lordosis are not acquired until later.

2. **ABCDE**

   The Ortolani test is employed in the neonatal period and in infancy to test for hip dislocation. In cases of established dislocation, there may be delayed walking, an abnormal gait, asymmetric skin creases in the groins and limited abduction. Ultrasound can be used to confirm the diagnosis and there is some evidence to support its use for mass screening for this condition in the newborn. Wherever possible, the diagnosis should be established early since, with greater delay, the risks of permanent joint deformity increase.

3. **BCD**

   Postural variations seen in childhood include: (1) bow legs in toddlers associated with internal tibial torsion; (2) knock knees presenting before adolescence; (3) out-toeing in infancy; and (4) most if not all cases of flat feet. Sternomastoid torticollis may present in the newborn and can resolve spontaneously. In children in whom there is progressive torticollis or who are over 2 years old, surgery is usually necessary. Scoliosis can be benign if it is non-progressive and mild. In cases where it is progressive or if the curve is more than 20°, specialist advice should be sought.

4. **BCDE**

   The majority (80%) of cases of scoliosis are idiopathic and a high proportion of these occur in adolescent girls. Identifiable causes may be classified into neuromuscular diseases, congenital spinal malformations and a small number of other disorders, including Marfan syndrome, in which there is ligamentous laxity.

5. **Regarding scoliosis:**
   A. if compensatory due to asymmetric leg length, the scoliosis will disappear on forward flexion.
   B. unilateral prominence of the ribs on forward flexion is a sign of scoliosis.
   C. the majority of cases develop in infancy.
   D. juvenile idiopathic scoliosis is more likely to cause permanent deformity than the adolescent form.
   E. 40% of adolescent idiopathic scoliosis cases will require surgery.

6. **The following observations are correctly paired with causes of a painful hip:**
   A. an age of 6 years in suspected slipped upper femoral epiphysis.
   B. a hip radiograph showing increased density of the femoral head in suspected slipped upper femoral epiphysis.
   C. male sex in suspected Perthes' disease.
   D. a history of systemic upset in suspected Perthes' disease.
   E. a normal ESR in suspected irritable hip (transient synovitis).

7. **At the time of presentation of juvenile chronic arthritis (JCA):**
   A. rheumatoid factor is positive in over half of all cases.
   B. in systemic JCA joint involvement may not occur until weeks or months after the onset of the illness.
   C. a fever of over 39°C is more suggestive of a diagnosis of septic arthritis than JCA.
   D. involvement of four or less joints suggests the pauciarticular form of the disease.
   E. hepatosplenomegaly and lymphadenopathy may lead to confusion with a diagnosis of acute leukaemia.

8. **Complications of juvenile chronic arthritis include:**
   A. violaceous rash over the eyes and bridge of the nose.
   B. uveitis.
   C. dysphagia due to oesophageal dysmotility.
   D. mandibular hypoplasia.
   E. atlanto-axial subluxation.

5. **B**

Scoliosis may be postural/compensatory or structural. Postural scoliosis disappears when the patient touches his toes. Compensatory scoliosis due to asymmetric leg length disappears when sitting. In idiopathic scoliosis there is rotation and curvature of the spine, causing a rib hump to develop. Infantile scoliosis is usually mild, non-progressive and treatment is rarely needed. The juvenile form is rare, but more often causes deformity. Adolescent idiopathic scoliosis is the commonest type, around 10% of cases will require surgery. Treatment is usually recommended if there is progression or a pronounced deformity of more than 25°.

6. **CE**

Perthes' disease occurs predominantly in boys aged 3–10 years who present with pain and limping. X-rays show decreased joint space with increased density of the femoral head, followed by destructive changes. Slipped upper femoral epiphysis is slightly commoner in peripubertal males. Hip X-rays show displacement of the epiphysis relative to the femoral neck. Irritable hip is also commoner in boys. There may be a mild fever, but not as marked as in septic arthritis, and the ESR and white cell count will be normal.

7. **BDE**

Non-articular features of systemic JCA include a swinging fever, rash, lymphadenopathy and hepatosplenomegaly, with little or no evidence of arthritis for weeks or months. In the pauciarticular form four or fewer joints are affected. The polyarticular form is often symmetrical, affecting large joints at first although small joints may be affected later. Most children with JCA do not have a positive rheumatoid factor.

8. **BDE**

Complications of JCA include growth impairment, uveitis leading to glaucoma and amyloidosis with renal impairment. The arthritis can cause permanent contractures and deformity. Atlanto-axial instability may predispose to cord compression. Inflammation in the temporo-mandibular joint can lead to mandibular hypoplasia. A violaceous rash is characteristic of dermatomyositis. Dysphagia occurs as a result of oesophageal dysmotility in scleroderma.

9. **When treating juvenile chronic arthritis:**
   A. bed rest is contra-indicated during acute exacerbations.
   B. paracetamol is an effective anti-inflammatory agent.
   C. oral corticosteroids are reserved for patients with disease refractory to first line therapy.
   D. prescription of alternate day corticosteroid therapy reduces toxicity.
   E. approximately half of all affected children will be left with long-term disability in adult life.

10. **Septic arthritis:**
    A. rarely occurs before 2 years of age.
    B. should be excluded by joint aspiration in all new cases where there is a single, inflamed joint with fever.
    C. can be excluded clinically if there is arthritis at more than one joint.
    D. presents in young children with apparent weakness of the affected limb.
    E. has a similar clinical presentation to osteomyelitis.

11. **When investigating and treating septic arthritis:**
    A. blood culture is valuable in identifying the infecting organism.
    B. the C-reactive protein (CRP) is unhelpful in monitoring the response to treatment.
    C. the majority of cases will not have radiological changes affecting the bone within 1 week of presentation.
    D. *Staphylococcus aureus* is a common causative pathogen.
    E. 10 days of antibiotic treatment is an adequate course of treatment to ensure elimination of the infection.

12. **Arthritis may occur in association with:**
    A. rotavirus gastroenteritis.
    B. haemophilia.
    C. ulcerative colitis.
    D. atopic dermatitis.
    E. psoriasis.

## 9. CD

Treatment of JCA involves physiotherapy and non-steroidal anti-inflammatory drugs. During acute exacerbations, bed rest allows inflammation to subside. Passive and then active physiotherapy prevents permanent joint contractures and muscle wasting. Paracetamol is a useful analgesic but has no anti-inflammatory effect. For patients who require long-term oral corticosteroid, alternate day therapy is effective in reducing the adverse effects. Over 80% of affected children will have little or no disability in adult life.

## 10. BDE

Septic arthritis can occur at any age but is commonest in children under 2 years of age. Consider the diagnosis in any child presenting with an acute arthritis of one joint, especially if there are signs of systemic illness. Most cases will require joint aspiration under anaesthetic to confirm the diagnosis. Bacteria usually spread to the joints via the bloodstream and up to 10% of cases of septic arthritis involve several joints. Children with septic arthritis are often reluctant to use the affected limb. The joint and the adjacent bone may be involved.

## 11. ACD

Septic arthritis is commonly associated with septicaemia and the responsible pathogen can often be identified in the blood-stream. Infection in a joint space can be difficult to eradicate. The C-reactive protein and erythrocyte sedimentation rate are often employed to monitor the response to treatment. Antibiotic treatment is often given for a prolonged course (e.g. 4 weeks). Destructive changes are unlikely to appear until 10 days or more after the onset of infection.

## 12. BCE

Causes of arthritis in childhood include juvenile chronic arthritis, ankylosing spondylitis and other connective tissue disorders. Arthritis is also seen in association with inflammatory bowel disease and psoriasis. Reactive arthritis follows infection with Salmonella, Shigella, Campylobacter and Yersinia. In haemophilia bleeding into the joint causes arthritis and, in some cases, a severe arthropathy with permanent impairment. Leukaemia may present with arthritis.

13. **The following criteria are used in making a diagnosis of Kawasaki disease:**
    A. bilateral non-purulent conjunctivitis.
    B. peeling of the skin on the palms or soles of the feet.
    C. arthritis at four or more joints.
    D. erythema and fissuring of the lips.
    E. biochemical evidence of hepatitis.

14. **In the management of Kawasaki disease:**
    A. echocardiography should be performed in all patients to identify coronary artery aneurysm.
    B. salicylate is effective for controlling fever and as an antithrombotic agent.
    C. methotrexate is useful in refractory cases.
    D. coronary artery surgery is required in around 10% of cases.
    E. intravenous gammaglobulin administered early in the course of the disease reduces the risk of coronary artery aneurysm formation.

15. **Regarding connective tissue diseases in childhood:**
    A. dermatomyositis carries a high mortality if untreated.
    B. infants born to mothers with systemic lupus erythematosus may be affected by congenital heart block.
    C. ankylosing spondylitis affects predominantly small joints of the distal limbs.
    D. dermatomyositis may cause a raised plasma creatine phosphokinase level.
    E. renal involvement in systemic lupus erythematosus is invariably benign.

16. **On examination of a 5-year-old child with a missed congenital dislocation of the hip:**
    A. there will be limited abduction of the hip on the affected side.
    B. there will be a fixed flexion deformity of the hip.
    C. there will be a positive Trendelenburg test.
    D. Ortolani's test will be positive.
    E. there will be true shortening of the affected leg.

**13. ABD**

Kawasaki disease is a clinical diagnosis and there is no definitive diagnostic investigation. The diagnosis is made when there is a fever over 38.5°C for 5 days or more, with four of the following criteria: (1) bilateral non-purulent conjunctivitis; (2) strawberry tongue and erythematous lips with fissuring; (3) cervical lymphadenopathy; (4) oedema and erythema of the hands or the feet, with peeling of the skin; and (5) polymorphous, non-vesicular rash.

**14. ABE**

When treating Kawasaki disease, salicylates are used as anti-inflammatory, anti-pyretic agents and later as anti-thrombotic agents to reduce the risk of coronary artery thrombosis. Gammaglobulin administered in the acute phase of the illness has been demonstrated to reduce the risk of coronary artery disease. Echocardiography may be used to screen for coronary artery involvement. Although up to 20% may develop coronary artery aneurysms, only a very few will develop myocardial ischaemia or infarction.

**15. ABD**

Dermatomyositis is manifested by a characteristic rash, muscle pain and weakness. It carries a significant mortality, although the use of corticosteroid therapy is generally effective. Babies born to mothers with systemic lupus may exhibit some features of the disease with a rash and heart block. In ankylosing spondylitis the arthritis predominantly affects the large joints and the spine. Renal involvement in SLE is a worrying complication.

**16. ABC**

There will be apparent shortening of the affected leg because the head of the femur lies above and behind the acetabulum. True leg length remains normal. There will be limited abduction of the hip. Once the lumbar lordosis has been eliminated by flexing the unaffected hip (Thomas's test), a fixed flexion deformity becomes obvious. Trendelenburg's sign – sagging of the pelvis when standing on the affected leg – is due to mechanical disadvantage of the muscles around the affected hip. The hip does not 'clunk' back into position after the first few weeks of life even if the hip remains dislocated; the signs become rather more subtle.

# Minitest 3

1. **The following are cyanotic congenital heart lesions:**
   A. persistent ductus arteriosus.
   B. truncus arteriosus.
   C. pulmonary atresia.
   D. coarctation of the aorta.
   E. transposition of the great vessels with patent foramen ovale.

2. **In scabies infection:**
   A. there is no involvement of the head or feet.
   B. the rash is intensely itchy.
   C. the rash appears within a few days of infection.
   D. the rash is vesicular.
   E. topical Malathion is the best treatment.

3. **In status asthmaticus the following features suggest that ventilation will be required:**
   A. an oxygen requirement of 40% to maintain oxygen saturation above 94%.
   B. agitation.
   C. drowsiness.
   D. arterial $PaCO_2$ 4.2 Kpa and pH 7.43.
   E. widespread wheezing on auscultation.

4. **Diplopia becomes worse:**
   A. if a child with a seventh nerve palsy looks down.
   B. if a child with a right third nerve palsy looks up and to the left.
   C. if a child with a left fourth nerve palsy closes the right eye.
   D. if a child with a left sixth nerve palsy looks to the left.
   E. the longer a paralytic squint goes untreated.

1. **BCE**

   Cyanotic heart disease is caused by *obstructive* lesions such as tricuspid atresia, pulmonary atresia, tetralogy of Fallot and transposition of the great vessels and total anomalous pulmonary venous drainage. Cyanosis also occurs when there is *mixing* of deoxygenated and oxygenated blood such as truncus arteriosus and single ventricle. In Ebstein's anomaly there is poorly contractile right ventricle, with resultant poor pulmonary blood flow and cyanosis.

2. **BDE**

   Scabies may involve the feet and head of babies, which is unusual in older patients. Scabies is intensely itchy. Family members are often infected. The rash does not appear until an allergic or inflammatory reaction occurs up to six weeks after the initial contact. Treatment is with Malathion preparation. The whole family should be treated. It will take some time for the lesions to subside after treatment.

3. **C**

   There are no absolute indications for ventilation in severe asthma. Management will differ depending on whether a patient is deteriorating or improving on treatment despite similar clinical findings and blood gas results. Hypoxia occurs early in asthma due to ventilation/perfusion mismatching. Hypoxia causes agitation and hyperventilation and results in a low $CO_2$ in mild or moderate asthma. Drowsiness in status asthmaticus indicates either exhaustion or a high $PCO_2$ which, if not quickly responding to treatment, may indicate a need for ventilation. Widespread wheezing suggests that there is still good ventilation – a silent chest is much more ominous.

4. **BD**

   Diplopia usually resolves when one eye is closed. Double vision is exacerbated by looking in the direction of action of the paralysed extraocular muscles. The facial nerve does not control eye movements. Over time, the image from a squinting eye will be suppressed and diplopia will disappear. Diplopia of recent onset is an important symptom and may indicate raised intracranial pressure, brain tumour, orbital tumour or, very rarely, myasthenia gravis.

5. **Coeliac disease:**
   A. causes symptoms within weeks of starting a gluten-containing diet.
   B. is commoner in children with IgA deficiency than in the general population.
   C. if asymptomatic, requires no treatment.
   D. affects the whole of the small bowel.
   E. affects 50% of first-degree relatives of an index case.

6. **Comparing the features of Turner syndrome and Noonan syndrome:**
   A. Turner syndrome is a recessive condition, while Noonan is dominantly inherited.
   B. Turner syndrome affects only females, while Noonan affects both sexes.
   C. Turner syndrome is associated with coarctation of the aorta and Noonan with pulmonary valve stenosis.
   D. both conditions are associated with severe learning disability.
   E. females with Turner syndrome are infertile, while fertility is normal in females with Noonan syndrome.

7. **Ambiguous genitalia in a newborn baby:**
   A. is associated with a risk of collapse towards the end of the first week of life.
   B. should result in rearing according to the genetic sex.
   C. if associated with a phallus and a normally positioned urethral meatus indicates the baby is genetically male.
   D. may result from excessive androgen production in fetal life.
   E. may result from lack of tissue response to testosterone.

8. **Causes of recurrent epistaxes in a 3-year-old boy include:**
   A. haemophilia A.
   B. regular use of paracetamol as an antipyretic.
   C. iron deficiency anaemia.
   D. von Willebrand's disease.
   E. local trauma.

5. **B**

Coeliac disease may present any time after the introduction of gluten into the diet or may remain asymptomatic. The small bowel may be affected in a patchy distribution. Untreated there is an increased risk of a small bowel lymphoma – a gluten-free diet should be continued for life. There is an increased incidence of coeliac disease in those with IgA deficiency. One must measure the IgA levels when measuring IgA antigliadin and anti-endomysial antibodies. Coeliac disease may occur in up to 15% of first-degree relatives of an index case.

6. **BCE**

Girls with Turner syndrome are infertile due to failure of development of the ovaries. Noonan syndrome children may have a Turner-like appearance, but have a normal karyotype. The precise genetic abnormality in Noonan syndrome is unknown, but may affect boys and girls and is often inherited in an autosomal dominant fashion. Noonan syndrome children often have significant learning disability, whereas in Turner syndrome there is a normal range of ability.

7. **ADE**

In adrenal hyperplasia the block in adrenal steroid production may result in salt loss and collapse during the first week of life. Genetic males should be raised as males only if there is an adequate phallus. Virilised females may have a hypertrophied clitoris surgically reduced. Excess androgens may virilise the female clitoris to appear as a normal penis, usually with no palpable gonads. Failure of tissue responsiveness to androgen results in a genetic male having female external genitalia but without ovaries or uterus – the testicular feminisation syndrome.

8. **DE**

Mucosal bleeds are not characteristic of haemophilia - soft tissue and joint bleeds are more typical. Paracetamol does not cause a bleeding tendency unless in overdose when haemorrhage may result from liver failure. Aspirin, not recommended for children, does reduce platelet stickiness and may predispose to mucosal bleeding. In von Willebrand's disease there is abnormal platelet function – epistaxes are common. Local trauma or nose picking is probably the commonest cause of nosebleeds.

9. **Ketotic hypoglycaemia is associated with:**
   A. newly diagnosed diabetes mellitus.
   B. starvation.
   C. fatty acid oxidation defects.
   D. hyperinsulinism.
   E. glycogen storage disorder type 1 (glucose-6-phosphatase deficiency).

10. **In otitis media:**
    A. pain is always present.
    B. wax will not obscure the tympanic membrane if a true otitis media is present.
    C. decongestants speed the resolution of the condition.
    D. the infection is always bacterial.
    E. penicillin V is the treatment of choice.

11. **The following problems are more likely to affect a preterm infant of 1.5 kg than a full-term infant of 1.5 kg:**
    A. birth asphyxia.
    B. intraventricular haemorrhage.
    C. meconium aspiration syndrome.
    D. hyperbilirubinaemia.
    E. polycythaemia.

12. **Unconjugated hyperbilirubinaemia:**
    A. will occur if a mother has blood group O-positive and her baby is group A-negative.
    B. is treated by phototherapy if the bilirubin rises above 250 μmol/L on day 3.
    C. should be treated by exchange transfusion if the bilirubin levels exceed 340 μmol/L at any time.
    D. is more common in infants of diabetic mothers than in equivalent gestation babies of healthy mothers.
    E. is an indication to discontinue breast feeding.

9. **BE**

Hypoglycaemia is an important diagnostic problem. The initial assessment must determine whether or not there is ketosis. Ketotic hypoglycaemia excludes abnormalities of fatty acid oxidation where few ketone bodies may be produced and excludes hyperinsulinaemic conditions. Ketosis develops where fat is the main metabolic substrate, usually when glycogen stores are depleted or not available. In the newly diagnosed diabetic there will be *hyper*glycaemia.

10. **All are false**

Pain is not always a feature of otitis media. Wax does not necessarily soften to reveal the inflamed tympanic membrane to the examining paediatrician! Decongestants have not been shown to be of any benefit in the treatment of acute otitis media. Viruses, Mycoplasma and bacteria may all cause ear infections. Bacterial infections causing otitis media include: Pneumococci, *H. influenzae*, *B. catarrhalis*, Group A Streptococci and Staphylococci.

11. **BD**

Premature infants are at risk of IRDS, bronchopulmonary dysplasia, intraventricular haemorrhage, jaundice, hypoglycaemia, hypothermia, necrotising enterocolitis, persistent ductus arteriosus, rickets and anaemia. Growth-retarded mature babies are at risk of birth asphyxia, meconium aspiration syndrome, hypothermia, hypoglycaemia and polycythaemia.

12. **D**

Approximately 15% of mothers who are blood group O have babies who are group A. This combination can lead to AO incompatibility. However, in most OA mother–baby combinations there is no red cell sensitisation. There is no absolute level of bilirubin above which phototherapy or an exchange transfusion should be started. Because insulin has a maturation-retarding effect (on liver glucuronyl transferase activity), infants of diabetic mothers are prone to more severe jaundice than the babies of non-diabetic mothers. Breast feeding may promote the enterohepatic circulation of bile and therefore tends to exaggerate and prolong jaundice. As breast milk jaundice is entirely benign, there is no indication to stop breast feeding.

13. **Ataxia may be associated with:**
    A. alcohol ingestion.
    B. optic nerve glioma.
    C. posterior fossa tumour.
    D. chickenpox.
    E. Guillain–Barré syndrome.

14. **The following diseases are examples of the hypersensitivity reactions given:**
    A. hay fever: type 4 – delayed hypersensitivity.
    B. post Streptococcal glomerulonephritis: type 3 – immune complex mediated.
    C. rhesus disease: type 2 – antibody-mediated cytotoxicity.
    D. anaphylaxis: type 1 – IgE mediated.
    E. Mantoux reaction: type 4 – delayed hypersensitivity.

15. **A 3-year-old child presents after a generalised convulsion lasting 3 min. When seen in the A&E department, his temperature is 38.5°C. He is playing happily with his mother and there are no abnormal physical signs:**
    A. a lumbar puncture should be performed immediately.
    B. an outpatient EEG should be performed.
    C. a white blood count of $20 \times 10^9$/L, with 80% neutrophils, would indicate the need for intravenous antibiotics while awaiting the results of an 'infection screen'.
    D. a blood glucose of 10 mmol/L would suggest developing diabetes mellitus.
    E. if there is a family history of fits, he should be started on oral sodium valproate.

16. **Intracranial calcification is associated with:**
    A. cutaneous depigmented patches.
    B. an ipsilateral scalp capillary haemangioma.
    C. a bitemporal visual field defect.
    D. chorioretinitis.
    E. short 4th and 5th metacarpals.

**13.  ACDE**
Ataxia, or unsteadiness on the feet, may result from: drug or alcohol ingestion; cerebellar disease caused by a tumour, hydrocephalus or infection. Chickenpox may be associated with a cerebellaritis; neuropathy affecting afferent or efferent nerves or spinal cord disease; and muscle weakness as seen in Guillain–Barré syndrome may result in loss of the fine motor control necessary for maintenance of balance.

**14.  BCDE**
Hay fever, urticaria and anaphylaxis are examples of type 1, IgE mediated responses.

**15.  None of these**
This child has had a typical febrile convulsion. Lumbar puncture should not be performed if there are no signs of meningeal irritation. There is no indication for an EEG or anticonvulsant treatment after a 'simple' febrile convulsion. Neutrophilia and hyperglycaemia are simply manifestations of a 'stress response' to the convulsion and require no treatment. Rectal diazepam is often supplied for administration at home in any further convulsion which did not resolve rapidly. If fits were recurring frequently, then short-term treatment with sodium valproate may be of benefit.

**16.  ABCDE – all true**
Depigmented skin patches are found in tuberose sclerosis – periventricular calcification is a feature. In Sturge–Weber syndrome there is a capillary haemangioma of the scalp. A capillary haemangioma in this site is associated with an underlying vascular malformation of the meninges and brain on the same side which may calcify. A bitemporal field defect may be caused by pressure on the optic chiasm from a craniopharyngioma which on X-ray may show as suprasellar calcification. Chorioretinitis is associated with infections, such as cytomegalovirus and toxoplasmosis, which may result in intracranial calcification. Short 4th and 5th metacarpals are seen in pseudohypoparathyroidism. Other features of this condition include intracranial and subcutaneous calcification, round face, short stature, obesity and mental retardation.

17. **Clinical features of rickets include:**
    A. frontal bossing of the skull.
    B. Harrison's sulcus.
    C. short stature.
    D. obesity.
    E. expansion of the ends of the long bones.

18. *Mycoplasma pneumoniae* **infection is associated with:**
    A. bilateral patchy chest X-ray consolidation.
    B. small basal pleural effusion.
    C. a pertussis-like coughing illness.
    D. an acute encephalopathy.
    E. Stevens–Johnson syndrome.

19. **Features of lead poisoning include:**
    A. cerebral oedema.
    B. constipation.
    C. anaemia.
    D. neuropathy.
    E. linear densities at the ends of long bones on X-ray.

20. **In congenital pyloric stenosis presenting with dehydration:**
    A. there will be a metabolic acidosis.
    B. there will be hypokalaemia.
    C. the diagnosis should be confirmed by barium meal.
    D. balloon dilatation of the pylorus is now the treatment of
       choice.
    E. 0.9% saline with added potassium is the intravenous fluid of
       choice.

17. **ABCE**

The clinical features of rickets result from poor bone miner-alisation and an overgrowth of osteoid. The bones are softer than normal. The skull bones may be thin (craniotabes). Fontanelle closure is delayed. There is bossing of the frontal bone. The antero-lateral chest wall may be indrawn to produce a Harrison's sulcus and the sternum may protrude (pigeon chest). The ends of the bones may be expanded at the wrist and ankles and at the end of the ribs (rachitic rosary). The bones of the legs may be bowed. Short stature is common.

18. **ABCDE – all of these**

Mycoplasma infection typically presents as a 'flu-like illness', followed by a troublesome cough which may mimic a *B. pertussis* infection. Chest X-rays show patchy consolidation and small basal effusions are common. Complications of Mycoplasma infections include: the development of cold agglutinins, erythema multiforme, Stevens–Johnson syndrome, acute encephalopathy and liver dysfunction.

19. **ABCDE – all of these**

Lead poisoning may cause a variety of GI symptoms, including abdominal pain and constipation. CNS involvement may present with recurrent vomiting, convulsions, raised intra-cranial pressure and coma, or with behavioural change and learning difficulties. A microcytic anaemia refractory to treat-ment may be seen. There may be basophilic stippling of the red cells. A neuropathy may occur in heavy metal, inorganic chemical and insecticide poisoning.

20. **BE**

In pyloric stenosis there is a hypochloraemic, hypokalaemic, hyponatraemic, metabolic alkalosis. The diagnosis is clinical but may be confirmed by ultrasound scan. Treatment is by surgical pyloromyotomy. Resuscitation with saline and potassium per-mits replacement of lost salts. The metabolic alkalosis will resolve so long as continued vomiting is avoided by stopping feeds.

# 9

## Infectious diseases and immunisation

1. **Tetanus:**
   A. immunisation should always be administered when a wound has been contaminated with soil.
   B. has been eradicated in the UK.
   C. prevention for unimmunised individuals may be achieved by maintaining high levels of immunity in the general population.
   D. immunisation is achieved by vaccinating with an attenuated strain of *Clostridium tetani*.
   E. immunity after a single immunisation is life-long.

2. **Immunisation against poliomyelitis:**
   A. in most individuals may be achieved by a single dose of vaccine.
   B. is performed by administration of a live attenuated virus.
   C. has globally eradicated wild poliomyelitis.
   D. can be complicated by clinical poliomyelitis when the virus is transmitted to unimmunised individuals.
   E. vaccination of contacts can be used to limit an outbreak of poliomyelitis.

3. **Measles vaccination:**
   A. is effective when administered to infants aged 3–6 months.
   B. may protect unvaccinated individuals if there is a high uptake of vaccine in the population.
   C. can prevent all cases of subacute sclerosing panencephalitis (SSPE).
   D. is contraindicated if there is a history of anaphylactic reaction to egg.
   E. has successfully reduced the number of deaths from measles in children who are suffering from leukaemia.

4. **The following vaccines contain live attenuated organisms:**
   A. rubella.
   B. diphtheria.
   C. mumps.
   D. Bacillus Calmette Guérin (BCG).
   E. whooping cough.

1. **All false**
   Tetanus occurs when a contaminated wound is infected by *Clostridium tetani*. It is the tetanus toxin which produces the clinical manifestations. Immunisation is achieved by injecting the modified exotoxin, not the organism. A high level of immunity in the population is of no benefit since there is no transmission between individuals. Over time, immunity declines; booster doses are after wound contamination in an individual who has not been immunised in the past 10 years.

2. **BDE**
   Poliomyelitis can be prevented by the injection of inactivated virus (three strains) but, in the UK, immunisation is performed by the administration of three doses of oral, live attenuated virus. A course of three doses is required for reliable immunisation. Polio remains endemic in some developing countries. Faecal excretion of the virus may occur for up to 6 weeks after vaccination. Infection acquired from recently immunised individuals accounts for one case of clinical poliomyelitis for every 2 million doses of oral vaccine. Such contact cases only occur in unimmunised individuals. Vaccination of contacts can prevent the spread of polio.

3. **BDE**
   Immunisation against measles may be unsuccessful during the first months of life because of passively transferred maternal antibody. A high rate of vaccination protects individuals who have been immunised and also limits spread through the population. SSPE may occur in vaccinated individuals but is more common after 'wild'-type virus. Measles virus cultured for immunisation is propagated in chicken embryo cell lines. Egg allergy is not a contraindication to immunisation unless there is a history of anaphylaxis.

4. **ACD**
   Live attenuated vaccines include poliomyelitis (oral form or Sabin), measles, mumps, BCG and rubella. Whooping cough and poliomyelitis vaccines (injectable form or Salk) contain inactivated organisms. Influenza, Haemophilus and Pneumococcal vaccines contain immunising components of the organisms. Tetanus and diphtheria vaccines contain toxin inactivated by formaldehyde, termed toxoid.

5. **The following are general contraindications to immunisation:**
   A. the presence of a coryzal illness without significant fever.
   B. a history of a fever up to 38°C following a previous dose of vaccine.
   C. high-dose corticosteroid therapy when using a live vaccine.
   D. a family history of febrile convulsions.
   E. a history of severe eczema.

6. **In the UK the schedule for childhood immunisation is as follows:**
   A. diphtheria/pertussis/tetanus vaccine at 2, 4 and 6 months of age.
   B. *Haemophilus influenzae* type B immunisation is at 18 months of age.
   C. rubella vaccine for both sexes at 12–15 months of age.
   D. booster doses of diphtheria, tetanus and polio at 4 years.
   E. BCG is given to neonates at risk of contact with tuberculosis.

7. **The following statements regarding immunisation are correct:**
   A. uptake rates of over 95% of the population are necessary to prevent the spread of infectious diseases through the community.
   B. rubella vaccine is administered because of the teratogenic potential of the virus; the illness itself carries minimal morbidity.
   C. *Haemophilus influenzae* type B vaccine offers effective protection against meningitis but not other forms of invasive Haemophilus infection.
   D. influenza vaccine offers around 70% protection to the prevailing strain of virus for around 1 year.
   E. pneumococcal vaccine is indicated in children prior to splenectomy.

8. **Immunisation is effective in:**
   A. preventing infection in infants following perinatal exposure from mothers who are carriers of Hepatitis B.
   B. protecting HIV-positive individuals against some infectious diseases.
   C. protecting against infection with respiratory syncytial virus.
   D. preventing varicella (chickenpox) in an infant whose mother develops the condition shortly before delivery.
   E. protecting premature infants only if delayed until 2 months after the expected date of delivery.

5.  **C**

    True contraindications to immunisation include acute illnesses, not minor infections without fever or systemic upset. A history of a previous *severe* local reaction, or a *severe* general reaction, within 72 hours of vaccination are valid contraindications. Live virus vaccines should not be administered to immuno-suppressed individuals, including patients receiving high-dose corticosteroid for more than 1 week within the past 3 months, those with malignancies and those receiving chemotherapy.

6.  **CDE**

    Diphtheria (D), Pertussis, Tetanus (T), Poliomyelitis (OPV) and *Haemophilus influenzae* (Hib) vaccines are given at 2, 3 and 4 months. Rubella vaccine was formerly given to girls at 10–14 years of age, but it is now given to all children as part of the MMR vaccine. DT & OPV vaccine booster doses are given before school entry. BCG vaccine is selectively administered to infants whose family members are in regular contact with areas where tuberculosis is endemic.

7.  **ABDE**

    Although individual recipients of vaccination benefit, a high rate of uptake in the community is more important from a public health perspective. Follow-up studies of Hib vaccination have shown dramatic reductions in the incidence of all forms of invasive disease. Viruses which have a high degree of antigenic variation are difficult to immunise against. Children who are asplenic are at increased risk of pneumococcal infection and should be vaccinated accordingly.

8.  **ABD**

    Administration of Hepatitis B vaccine and specific immuno-globulin to babies at risk soon after birth reduces the risk of vertical transmission of infection. A varicella vaccine is not yet available for routine use. Infants born to mothers with acute VZ infection can be protected (passive immunity) by the admin-istration of specific immunoglobulin (VZIG). In general, live vaccines are contraindicated in immunocompromised patients, but HIV-positive individuals may safely receive them but should not receive BCG. Prematurely born infants can be effectively immunised according to the standard schedule. There is no RSV vaccine in use at present.

9. **Contraindications to the administration of the pertussis vaccine include:**
   A. a family history of epilepsy.
   B. the presence of cerebral palsy.
   C. a history of a previous episode of whooping cough.
   D. a history of cot death in a sibling.
   E. a history of irritability lasting 1 hour following a previous dose of vaccine.

10. **In measles:**
    A. virtually all affected individuals suffer respiratory tract symptoms.
    B. giant cell pneumonia is confined to immunosuppressed children.
    C. encephalitis carries a significant mortality even in developed countries.
    D. fever rarely exceeds 38°C.
    E. acute airway obstruction is a recognised complication.

11. **Chickenpox:**
    A. may be contracted by contact with fluid from vesicles.
    B. is infectious for 7 days after all vesicles have crusted over.
    C. is potentially life-threatening in children receiving cancer chemotherapy.
    D. encephalitis is generally benign and, in most cases, resolves completely.
    E. is a recognised cause of congenital malformation when the mother is affected in the first 5 months of pregnancy.

12. **During infection with mumps:**
    A. serum amylase is often elevated.
    B. parotid swelling is invariably bilateral.
    C. asymptomatic meningoencephalitis occurs in more than 50% of cases.
    D. orchitis develops in 80% of prepubertal males.
    E. no clinical signs may be apparent.

9. **All false**

Anxieties about the possibility that the pertussis vaccine could cause an encephalopathic illness and, in some cases, permanent brain damage led to a significant reduction in the uptake of the vaccine in the past. There have now been several studies completed which have examined this problem; if the pertussis vaccine does have the potential to cause encephalopathy, the incidence of this complication is extremely low and is certainly less common than neurological complications of pertussis disease. Current contraindications for pertussis are therefore no different from the general contraindications for other vaccines.

10. **ACE**

Respiratory tract involvement is universal in measles causing laryngitis and tracheobronchitis. Measles causes a high fever and systemic upset even in those who are spared complications. Although measles carries a high mortality in the developing world, in the developed world too encephalitis causes death in around 10% of affected individuals. Giant cell pneumonia is a fatal form of pneumonia which occurs predominantly in children with immune deficiency.

11. **ACDE**

Varicella virus is spread by respiratory tract droplets or by contact with fluid from vesicles which contain large amounts of virus. Affected individuals cease to be infectious once the last crop of vesicles have dried. Chickenpox is generally a benign illness but is potentially dangerous to the immunosuppressed and to the fetus. Complications such as encephalitis and pneumonia resolve in most cases. Similarly, most cases of intrauterine infection with varicella do not cause fetal damage, but occasionally lead to limb hypoplasia, microcephaly, cataracts, growth retardation and skin scarring.

12. **ACE**

Mumps parotitis or pancreatitis can both cause increased serum amylase. There is a CSF pleocytosis in up to 60% of cases, although only 10% suffer symptomatic meningitis. Orchitis is uncommon in prepubertal males. Subclinical infection is common.

**13. Infection with Herpes simplex virus:**
  A. in young children can cause a severe stomatitis.
  B. carries a high mortality if associated with encephalitis.
  C. in a child with eczema should be treated promptly with acyclovir.
  D. in the oral cavity is unlikely to resolve without intravenous acyclovir.
  E. which recurs is usually due to reinfection from a close family member.

**14. Human immunodeficiency virus infection in children:**
  A. in most cases is due to administration of contaminated blood products.
  B. may present with *Pneumocystis pneumoniae* infection in a previously asymptomatic child.
  C. may present with neurological signs in the absence of immunodeficiency.
  D. is more likely to present with recurrent bacterial infections than in adults.
  E. may be acquired by breast feeding from an infected mother.

**15. A comatose, 6-year-old girl is admitted to hospital with signs and symptoms suggestive of bacterial meningitis:**
  A. antibiotic therapy should be commenced after the sensitivities of the infecting organism are known.
  B. the responsible organism is most likely to be Group B Streptococcus.
  C. a lumbar puncture should be performed promptly to identify the pathogen and confirm the diagnosis.
  D. cerebral oedema is a likely explanation for her coma.
  E. persistent fever after several days of appropriate antibiotic therapy may be associated with the presence of a subdural effusion.

13. **ABC**

Primary infection with Herpes simplex type 1 causes a painful gingivostomatitis, usually in young children. Herpes has the potential to cause life-threatening illness – e.g. Herpes skin infection in a child with eczema, encephalitis, infection in an immunosuppressed individual or in a newborn. Following primary infection, the virus remains latent in the host but may periodically cause stomatitis or cold sore.

14. **BCDE**

Most HIV infection in children results from vertical transmission from an infected mother. Symptomatic disease presents with infections typical of immunocompromised individuals, but bacterial infection is more common in affected infants than in adults, probably because of the infant's relative immunoglobulin deficiency. HIV can also cause direct injury to various organ systems and some infants present with developmental delay, regression or motor signs, caused by HIV encephalopathy.

15. **DE**

In suspected cases of bacterial meningitis, antibiotic therapy should be commenced promptly to cover the likely pathogens. In older children the commonest organisms are *Neisseria meningitidis*, *Streptococcus pneumoniae* and *Haemophilus influenzae*, although the incidence of the latter is falling with the use of the Hib vaccine. Cerebral oedema is a common important complication of meningitis. If there is alteration in conscious level, lumbar puncture should be deferred because of the risk of coning. A minority of cases are complicated by subdural effusions which can present with persistent fever.

16. **An 18-month-old boy rapidly becomes unwell with a fever and a purpuric rash. Meningococcal disease is suspected:**
    A. rapid onset suggests a worse prognosis.
    B. his general practitioner should administer an intramuscular dose of antibiotic before sending him to hospital.
    C. death is likely to result from complications of meningitis.
    D. close family contacts need treatment with prophylactic oral antibiotics.
    E. the same clinical picture could be caused by *Haemophilus influenzae.*

17. **When interpreting the results of a lumbar puncture in a 10-year-old:**
    A. normal cerebrospinal fluid (CSF) contains up to $10 \times 10^6$ polymorphs per litre.
    B. a cell count of $10 \times 10^6$ polymorphs per litre excludes a viral meningitis.
    C. a CSF glucose concentration of less than 40% of the blood glucose value is suggestive of bacterial meningitis.
    D. after antibiotics have been administered, CSF examination is of no benefit in diagnosing bacterial meningitis.
    E. tuberculous meningitis is associated with an elevated CSF lymphocyte count.

18. **Infectious mononucleosis:**
    A. is most commonly transmitted by infected saliva.
    B. can be diagnosed clinically with confidence in most cases.
    C. causes hepatitis in up to half of cases.
    D. can cause life-threatening upper airway obstruction.
    E. is effectively treated using Ampicillin.

**16.  ABDE**

Meningococcal disease can cause septicaemia or meningitis, or both. Meningitis can usually be cured, whereas the septicaemic illness carries a significant mortality. Rapid onset of illness is one of a number of poor prognostic features. If the diagnosis is suspected, a dose of intramuscular antibiotic should be administered immediately. Close contacts of an affected individual are at increased risk of developing symptomatic infection and should be treated with prophylactic oral antibiotic. The clinical features described are typical of meningococcal infection but occasionally an identical picture is caused by Haemophilus or other bacteria.

**17.  CE**

Normal CSF contains up to $5 \times 10^6$ white cells per litre which are predominantly lymphocytes. Any increase in polymorphs may indicate bacterial meningitis, although in most cases polymorph counts will be in the 100s or 1000s. Although viral meningitis is typically characterised by an increase in lymphocytes, there may be an increase in polymorphs at the onset of the infection. Prior administration of antibiotic may prevent the culture of bacteria from the CSF, but culture of viruses, identification of bacterial antigen by latex agglutination and differential cell counts can still be useful.

**18.  ACD**

Infectious mononucleosis is caused by the Epstein–Barr virus, in most cases transmitted by contact with infected saliva. If pharyngitis, lymphadenopathy and splenomegaly are present, then the diagnosis can be made with some confidence but, in many cases, the symptoms and signs are non-specific. Up to 50% of cases have biochemical evidence of hepatitis; rarely there may be more serious complications of clinical hepatitis, splenic rupture, encephalitis or upper airway obstruction due to massive tonsillar enlargement. Treatment is supportive. The viral aetiology means that antibiotics are of no benefit and Ampicillin given during the illness is known to cause a non-specific macular rash.

# 10

## Immunology and allergy

1. **Regarding the early immunological development of the infant:**
    A. in the newborn, there are significant quantities of circulating IgM.
    B. IgG is actively transported across the placenta.
    C. in the normal newborn neutrophil function is reduced.
    D. a large thymus gland, detected on chest X-ray, is a normal finding.
    E. circulating immunoglobulin levels will have reached normal adult levels by 6 months.

2. **The following indicate a need for investigation of immune function:**
    A. several episodes of upper respiratory tract infection and gastroenteritis in the space of 1 year.
    B. two episodes of bacterial meningitis.
    C. absence of tonsils in the 2nd year of life.
    D. a history of chronic diarrhoea and oral candidiasis.
    E. a history of a first-cousin marriage in the parents of a child with recurrent pneumonia.

3. **The following infections are appropriately paired with a relevant immune deficiency:**
    A. recurrent pneumococcal infection and complement deficiency.
    B. recurrent viral infection and hypogammaglobulinaemia.
    C. cutaneous abscesses and IgA deficiency.
    D. osteomyelitis and chronic granulomatous disease.
    E. disseminated viral infections and T-cell deficiency.

4. **Atopy:**
    A. affects around 1 in 5 individuals.
    B. can be prevented by exclusive breast feeding during the 1st year.
    C. is characterised by reduced circulating IgE.
    D. is familial.
    E. is excluded if skin tests to four common allergens are negative.

1. **BCD**
   During the last trimester of pregnancy, there is active transport of IgG across the placenta. At birth a baby's IgM and IgA levels will be extremely low. There is a decline in IgG level during the first 9 months, but a rise to adult levels at around 18 months. The newborn's risk of infection is increased by reduced neutrophil function, reduced complement levels and lack of immunological 'memory' from previous exposure to pathogens. The thymus is large in early infancy.

2. **BCDE**
   Healthy children have frequent infections in the first few years of life. The possibility of an immune deficiency should be considered if there is: (1) recurrent severe infections (pneumonia, meningitis, etc.); (2) infections with organisms of low virulence should raise the suspicion; (3) persistent diarrhoea or oral candidiasis; (4) absence of lymphoid or thymic tissue; or (5) a history of other affected siblings – most immune deficiencies have an autosomal recessive inheritance and are more common in consanguineous marriages.

3. **ADE**
   Immunoglobulin deficiency (hypogammaglobulinaemia) and abnormality of neutrophil function (e.g. chronic granulomatous disease) or neutrophil numbers are likely to present in infancy with recurrent bacterial infections. An exception to this is IgA deficiency which is often asymptomatic. Complement deficiency is associated with recurrent bacterial infection, particularly with encapsulated bacteria. Deficiencies of T-lymphocyte number or function (DiGeorge syndrome, severe combined immunodeficiency) predispose to bacterial infection but are more commonly linked to potentially life-threatening viral and fungal infections.

4. **AD**
   Atopy is common, affecting 10–20% of individuals. It is suggested that limiting allergen exposure in infancy can prevent development of atopic disease, but trials of allergen avoidance generally show delayed onset rather than prevention of allergic disease. There is no diagnostic test for atopy, but elevated circulating IgE, and eosinophil count and positive skin tests to common allergens (pollen, cat, dog, aspergillus fungus, house dust mite), are supportive evidence.

5. **Perennial rhinitis:**
   A. affects children more commonly than adults.
   B. is associated with the presence of a transverse nasal crease.
   C. may be confused with persistent upper respiratory tract infection.
   D. is characterised by habitual mouth breathing.
   E. responds to topical nasal corticosteroid in the majority of cases.

6. **In children with food allergies:**
   A. a negative skin test excludes the diagnosis.
   B. the commonest allergens are vegetables and fruit.
   C. most allergies will resolve before 5 years of age.
   D. a delayed hypersensitivity reaction is normally associated with a positive skin test to that food.
   E. a diagnosis may be made if there is a convincing history, even without supportive investigations.

7. **In many cases of atopic dermatitis:**
   A. remission can be achieved by strict dietary exclusions.
   B. there is an increase in circulating IgE.
   C. skin testing can be used to identify exacerbating factors in the diet.
   D. measles immunisation should be omitted because of the increased risk of egg hypersensitivity.
   E. factors other than allergy are important in causing worsening disease.

8. **An anaphylactic reaction:**
   A. is an example of type 1 hypersensitivity.
   B. should be treated with subcutaneous atropine.
   C. causing facial swelling should be treated by fluid restriction.
   D. may present with acute onset wheeze.
   E. is a recognised complication of radiographic contrast media.

5. **BCDE**

Perennial rhinitis is an atopic condition characterised by nasal mucosal oedema and hypersecretion leading to nasal obstruction and discharge, sneezing, snoring and mouth breathing. Parents may report that the child 'has a permanent cold'. Repeated upward rubbing of an itchy nose may cause a transverse crease on the nose. Perennial rhinitis is commoner than seasonal rhinitis before adolescence. Either topical sodium cromoglycate or corticosteroids are effective treatments.

6. **CE**

Food allergies may be immediate (occurring within 2 hours of ingestion) and characterised by vomiting, urticaria and facial swelling. Delayed reactions occur up to 48 hours after ingestion with vomiting, diarrhoea and sometimes with exacerbation of eczema. In delayed hypersensitivity the immunological mechanism is uncertain and testing is not possible. In food allergy the history is central to the diagnosis and is confirmed by challenge with the suspected food – allergy testing often adds little. The commonest food allergies are to milk, egg and peanuts. Food allergies usually present in the first 3 years and resolve within 2–5 years.

7. **BE**

In atopic dermatitis IgE mediated allergic reactions play an important part but other factors such as delayed hypersensitivity, other immunological abnormalities, environmental factors (humidity, temperature) and infection all contribute. Improvement is achieved in a minority of patients by dietary restriction, and skin tests are often unhelpful in identifying which foods may be responsible. Even in children who are allergic to egg, a previous anaphylactic reaction, which would contraindicate the measles vaccine, is exceedingly rare.

8. **ADE**

Anaphylactic reactions are type 1 hypersensitivity reactions which present within 1–2 hours of exposure to the allergen with wheeze, stridor and circulatory failure. Treatment involves adrenaline injection, oxygen, bronchodilators, steroids and antihistamine. Circulatory failure is treated by volume expansion and vasoconstricting drugs. Recognised precipitants of anaphylaxis include antibiotics, foods, radiographic contrast media and insect stings.

9. **Type 1 hypersensitivity reactions:**
   A. to an antibiotic are unlikely to occur if there has been no reaction to a previous course of the same drug.
   B. are IgA mediated.
   C. are commoner in individuals with a family history of allergy.
   D. are unaffected by antihistamines.
   E. is an inherited disorder with 100% concordance in identical twins.

**9. C**

Type 1 hypersensitivity reactions occur following interaction of an allergen with specific IgE antibody on the surfaces of mast cells and basophils. This causes release of inflammatory mediators (including histamines) from these cells, resulting in the development of symptoms. Atopy is the predisposition to develop such reactions and is an inherited condition, although the genetics are incompletely understood. Clinical allergic disease results from an interaction between the susceptible individual and environmental factors. Thus there is only a 50% concordance in identical twins. Repeated exposure to the antigen is required. Drug allergies may occur at any time following introduction of a drug. Antihistamines are effective in reducing symptoms in a variety of atopic disorders.

# 11

## Oncology

1. **Children with the following genetic disorders have an increased risk of malignancy:**
   A. ataxia telangiectasia.
   B. neurofibromatosis type 1.
   C. congenital hemihypertrophy.
   D. Down syndrome.
   E. achondroplasia.

2. **Cancer in children:**
   A. has an overall incidence of 1 in 10 000.
   B. is the third commonest cause of death in childhood.
   C. has a survival rate of 30%.
   D. is associated with an increased incidence if a parent suffers from malignancy.
   E. most commonly takes the form of leukaemia.

3. **Clinical findings in a child with newly diagnosed leukaemia include:**
   A. bruising.
   B. anaemia.
   C. splenomegaly.
   D. bone pain.
   E. lymphoblasts on a peripheral blood film.

4. **Good prognostic features of acute lymphoblastic leukaemia (ALL) at presentation include:**
   A. high white cell count.
   B. female sex.
   C. age less than 1 year.
   D. testicular enlargement.
   E. lymphoblasts in the cerebrospinal fluid.

1. **ABCD**

   In at least 200 genetic disorders there is an increased risk of neoplasia. In ataxia telangiectasia there is DNA repair defect. There is progressive ataxia, telangiectasia and repeated respiratory tract infections. Neurofibromatosis has a moderate risk of intracranial neoplasia, neuroblastoma and phaeochromocytoma. Congenital hemihypertrophy is associated with an increased risk of Wilms tumours, hepatoblastomas and adrenal carcinomas. Children with Down syndrome have a 15% chance of developing leukaemia. In achondroplasia there is no increased incidence of neoplasia.

2. **BDE**

   The incidence of cancer in childhood is 1.36/1000 live births. Outside the newborn period cancer is the third commonest cause of death after accidents and congenital anomalies. The commonest childhood cancer is leukaemia, which constitutes one-third of all childhood malignancies. The cure rates are now 60–70% overall – a dramatic improvement over the past 20 years. There is an increased incidence noted in certain 'cancer families', related to a genetic predisposition.

3. **ABCDE – all true**

   In leukaemia the bone marrow is almost fully replaced by malignant cells, so other cell precursors are reduced. Thrombocytopenia may present with easy bruising, bleeding and anaemia. The diagnosis is confirmed by bone marrow aspirate, although blasts or malignant cells are often seen in the peripheral blood film. The spleen may be enlarged if it is infiltrated by leukaemic cells. Skeletal bones and marrow are classically involved and children will often complain of bone pain.

4. **B**

   At presentation disease is classified as standard or high risk. This affects the child's long-term prognosis and also determines the most suitable treatment. Good prognostic features are female sex, Caucasian, age between 1 and 10 years, low white cell count and the common type ALL. Involvement of CNS or testicles at diagnosis carries poorer prognosis because these areas are relatively impermeable to chemotherapy and so can be the site of relapse.

5. **In the current treatment of acute lymphoblastic leukaemia:**
   A. the cure rate is 40%.
   B. the standard duration of treatment is 6 months.
   C. all children receive central nervous system directed therapy.
   D. the aim is to induce remission within 4 weeks of treatment.
   E. alopecia is preventable.

6. **Presenting features of brain tumours include:**
   A. cranial nerve palsy.
   B. visual field defect.
   C. acute torticollis.
   D. weight loss.
   E. delayed puberty.

7. **Radiotherapy:**
   A. causes pubertal delay.
   B. causes precocious puberty.
   C. causes cognitive problems.
   D. burns the skin in the treatment field.
   E. is first-line treatment for all brain tumours.

8. **Neuroblastoma:**
   A. may spontaneously regress without treatment.
   B. commonly presents with abdominal mass.
   C. prognosis is determined by age at presentation.
   D. may be detected by measuring urinary catecholamines.
   E. commonly presents at stage IV.

5. **CD**

   Currently the expected cure rate is 70%. Standard treatment aims to achieve remission after 4 weeks of chemotherapy (the induction), that is a reduction in tumour bulk from $10^{12}$ to $10^{10}$ cells. Treatment then continues for a total of 2 years with continuing chemotherapy. All children receive CNS-directed therapy, with intrathecal injections, because of the known risk of CNS relapse. Unfortunately, hair loss is unavoidable and occurs after episodes of intensive treatment.

6. **ABCDE**

   Brain tumours present in a large variety of ways. The classical signs of raised intracranial pressure – headaches, early morning vomiting – may either not be present or be attributed to other causes. Cranial nerve palsies may originate from compression of brain stem as in pontine gliomas. Visual field defects occur in craniopharyngiomas with destruction of the optic chiasm. Acute torticollis occurs in cerebellar tumours. Weight loss occurs in diencephalic syndrome. Delayed puberty occurs in tumours involving the hypothalamus and pituitary.

7. **ACD**

   Radiotherapy causes cell death. The pituitary gland is very sensitive and growth hormone deficiency is inevitable above a certain dose. Pubertal delay is also very common if there is radiotherapy to the gonads. Radiotherapy may burn the skin within the treatment field, but this recovers after completion. Cranial irradiation is known to cause cognitive problems, but must be used for treatment of some brain tumours which are not sensitive to chemotherapy and cannot be excised. In very young children radiotherapy is avoided whenever possible because of the damage to the developing brain.

8. **ACDE**

   Neuroblastoma is a heterogeneous tumour. It can present below the age of 1 year and spontaneously regress. However, they usually present at stage IV with bone marrow metastases. The commonest presenting symptoms are malaise, weight loss and bone pain. The prognosis is very poor for children older than 2 years. Elevation of urine catecholamines is diagnostic but not present in all cases.

9. **Wilms tumour (nephroblastoma):**
   A. presents with haematuria in 75% of cases.
   B. is associated with congenital abnormalities.
   C. may present with heart failure.
   D. metastasises to the lung.
   E. has a survival rate of 50%.

10. **Cervical lymphadenopathy is present in:**
   A. 20% of cases of Hodgkin's disease at diagnosis.
   B. 50–75% of cases of infectious mononucleosis.
   C. all cases of acute lymphoblastic leukaemia.
   D. atypical mycobacterium infection of cervical glands.
   E. 10% of cases of toxoplasmosis.

9. **BCD**

Wilms tumour usually presents in a well child incidentally noted to have an abdominal mass. There is an increased risk associated with certain congenital abnormalities – hemihypertrophy, aniridia and urogenital abnormalities – and these children should be monitored. Wilms tumours are known to metastasise along the inferior vena cava and can reach the right ventricle causing heart failure. They also metastasise to the lungs and may be present at diagnosis or relapse. The cure rate is a great success of paediatric oncology, with 90% surviving.

10. **BD**

Cervical lymphadenopathy is a common clinical finding usually related to minor infections and resolves quickly. If persistent, other causes are considered. Infectious causes include infectious mononucleosis, atypical mycobacterium and toxoplasmosis which is said to mimic Hodgkin's disease in presentation. Lymph node involvement is the most common feature of acquired toxoplasmosis. 80% of cases of Hodgkin's disease present with cervical lymphadenopathy. Acute lymphoblastic leukaemia does not typically involve cervical lymph nodes.

# 12

# Haematology

1. **Haemoglobin:**
   A. is present in blood cells by the 14th day after gestation.
   B. is predominantly produced in the liver at term.
   C. at term is mainly fetal haemoglobin.
   D. production increases after delivery.
   E. concentration at birth is 10–12 g/dl.

2. **Regarding anaemia in children:**
   A. iron deficiency is the most common cause.
   B. mucosal pallor is a useful clinical sign.
   C. a macrocytic blood film indicates iron deficiency anaemia.
   D. blood transfusions are standard treatment.
   E. occurs in less than 5% of the population.

3. **Idiopathic thrombocytopenia purpura:**
   A. results from decreased platelet production.
   B. classically presents with acute blood loss.
   C. requires urgent treatment to prevent intracranial haemorrhage.
   D. should be confirmed by bone marrow aspirate if there is no response to steroid therapy.
   E. is preceded by a viral URTI in more than 60% of cases.

4. **In a child presenting with acute haemolysis due to an inherited haemolytic anaemia:**
   A. anaemia is present only after complete failure of haemopoiesis.
   B. the plasma conjugated bilirubin level is elevated.
   C. reticulocyte count will be less than 1%.
   D. plasma haptoglobin will be elevated.
   E. there is excess urinary urobilinogen.

1. **AC**
   Haemoglobin can be detected by the 14th day in primitive circulation. The fetal liver is the main producer of haemoglobin in mid-trimester but by term the bone marrow is the main site; however, the main type is still fetal haemoglobin. The average haemoglobin concentration is 18 g/dl, and after delivery there is virtual cessation of erythropoiesis until 3 months old, when erythropoietin levels increase and Hb production is predominantly adult-type haemoglobin.

2. **AB**
   The commonest cause of anaemia is iron deficiency. This is due to poor diet and often excessive milk intake, which has low Fe content. The clinical features of anaemia in children are minimal and mucosal pallor is the most reliable. Fe deficiency is characterised by a hypochromic, microcytic picture. After taking a dietary history, treatment for anaemia is with an iron preparation for 2–3 months. A blood transfusion is rarely indicated. Iron deficiency is indeed common; in some populations it has been quoted as high as 30%.

3. **E**
   In ITP massive numbers of platelets are produced but rapidly consumed by an immune-mediated process thought to be triggered by viral exposure. It classically presents with purpuric spots but can present with blood loss from the GI tract or as epistaxis. It very rarely results in intracranial haemorrhage. Treatment with steroids is only considered if there is persistent low levels of platelets as length and degree of thrombocytopenia does correlate with increased morbidity. Steroid therapy must be preceded by bone marrow aspirate to exclude leukaemia.

4. **E**
   The bone marrow capacity can increase eightfold before anaemia is evident. The haemolysis may be detected by other indices. Haemolysis results in an increased red cell turnover and is accompanied by a high reticulocyte count. The increased cell destruction results in elevated plasma unconjugated bilirubin and therefore excess urinary urobilinogen. Haptoglobin binds to free plasma haemoglobin and is thus consumed in haemolysis.

5. **In thalassaemia:**
   A. the diagnosis is made on the blood film.
   B. the anaemia is due to deficiency in synthesis of globin chains.
   C. the anaemia is mainly due to haemolysis.
   D. splenectomy is treatment of choice at diagnosis.
   E. the serum iron level is normal at diagnosis.

6. **The clinical picture of B-thalassaemia major:**
   A. presents at birth.
   B. is characterised by iron deficiency anaemia.
   C. may initially present as failure to thrive.
   D. includes hepatosplenomegaly.
   E. is confirmed if investigation reveals markedly raised HbF on electrophoresis.

7. **In sickle cell disease:**
   A. there is an abnormality of the red cell membrane.
   B. symptoms result from tissue infarction.
   C. there is some protection against *Plasmodium falciparum* malaria.
   D. sickling crises can be prevented by morphine.
   E. sickling risk can be reduced by exchange transfusion.

8. **Haemophilia A:**
   A. is the commonest inherited bleeding disorder.
   B. inheritance is autosomal dominant with variable penetrance.
   C. severity is determined by level of factor VIIIc.
   D. is treated with factor VIII given by intramuscular injection.
   E. is no longer treated with prophylactic factor VIII because of HIV risk.

5. **BE**

   In thalassaemia there is defective synthesis of the alpha or beta globin chains resulting in anaemia. Accumulation of the abnormal haemoglobin results in haemolysis, which exacerbates the anaemia but is not the basic cause. The diagnosis is confirmed on Hb electrophoresis. Extramedullary haemopoiesis causes splenomegaly, resulting in further secondary hypersplenism and haemolysis, which may necessitate splenectomy. Prior to transfusion treatment, the serum iron levels are normal. Transfusion siderosis may develop in teenage life.

6. **CDE**

   Symptoms do not usually present until the first few years of life. At birth Hb electrophoresis is not diagnostic because of the high levels of HbF. Persisting elevation of HbF beyond 6 months is diagnostic. Clinical presentation is with failure to thrive, repeated infection, severe anaemia, or evidence of extramedullary haemopoiesis with splenomegaly and bone expansion.

7. **BE**

   Sickle cell disease (HbS) is due to alteration in the amino acid sequence of the beta-haemoglobin chain. The sickle haemoglobin may crystallise, forming sickle-shaped red cells that block capillaries, causing tissue infarction. Hypoxia and infection may trigger a sickling crisis. Treatment cannot prevent sickling, although exacerbating factors may be minimised. Management of sickling crises includes analgesia and hydration. Exchange transfusion reduces sickle cell numbers – e.g. prior to elective surgery. In sickle cell trait, the HbS heterozygous state, there is a degree of protection against *P. falciparum* malaria.

8. **AC**

   Haemophilia A is an X-linked recessive condition. It is the commonest inherited bleeding disorder and is caused by low levels of factor VIIIc – i.e. levels less than 2% of normal cause severe haemophilia. Factor VIII is given by intravenous injection. Haemophiliacs should never receive intramuscular injections. Prophylactic factor VIII is widely used. Recombinant factor VIII is not widely available. All donors are screened for HIV. A large number of haemophiliacs have died of HIV disease.

9. **Hazards of blood transfusion include:**
   A. haemosiderosis.
   B. circulatory failure.
   C. hypokalaemia.
   D. disseminated intravascular coagulation.
   E. cytomegalovirus infection.

10. **Neutropenia:**
   A. is defined as a circulatory count less than $5 \times 10^9/L$.
   B. increases susceptibility to viral infections.
   C. can be caused by cotrimoxazole.
   D. may be cyclical.
   E. may be a complication of folate deficiency.

9. **ABDE**

Blood transfusions should not be given without careful consideration. There is a risk of transmitted infection with blood-borne viruses such as HIV, Hepatitis C and CMV. Transfusion reactions can cause disseminated intravascular coagulation. Electrolyte imbalances, especially hyperkalaemia, may occur after large transfusions. Excess fluid load may precipitate cardiac failure. Repeated transfusions in haemolytic disorders lead to excess iron load which may require chelation treatment as in thalassaemia.

10. **CDE**

Neutropenia is defined as a circulating neutrophil count less than $1 \times 10^9$. It particularly increases the risk of bacterial infections, and patients may present with recurrent septicaemia. It can be caused by a variety of drugs, including cotrimoxazole. Folate deficiency decreases marrow ability to produce neutrophils. It is also known to occur in certain people cyclically – known as cyclical neutropenia – and during these troughs they are at risk of sepsis.

# 13

# Gastroenterology

1. **Polyhydramnios during the last trimester of pregnancy is associated with the following conditions which affect the fetus:**
   A. duodenal atresia.
   B. congenital myopathy.
   C. renal agenesis.
   D. oesophageal atresia.
   E. posterior urethral valves.

2. **Cleft palate:**
   A. is associated with recurrent secretory otitis media.
   B. is inherited as an autosomal dominant characteristic.
   C. is always associated with a cleft lip.
   D. causes feeding difficulties in infancy.
   E. should cause no further problems after surgical repair.

3. **Pierre Robin syndrome – micrognathia and central cleft palate – is associated with:**
   A. macroglossia.
   B. upper airway obstruction.
   C. feeding difficulty.
   D. trisomy 21.
   E. pulmonary hypertension.

4. **Causes of recurrent oral candidiasis in infancy include:**
   A. hypothyroidism.
   B. use of a comforter or dummy.
   C. thymic aplasia.
   D. inadequate hygiene.
   E. administration of antibiotics.

1.  **ABD**
    Over the last trimester of pregnancy, the fetus must be able to swallow amniotic fluid which is then absorbed from the gut. Fetal urine makes a large contribution to amniotic fluid volume over the last trimester of pregnancy. Any disturbance of swallowing or passage of fluid into the small bowel will result in polyhydramnios. Any reduction in the production of urine or obstruction to flow will result in oligohydramnios.

2.  **AD**
    Eustachian tube dysfunction is a common cause of chronic conductive hearing loss in young children with cleft palate. Cleft palate may occur with or without an associated cleft lip. The risk of recurrence does not follow simple Mendelian inheritance and is increased to 1:50 with an affected sibling, and 1:6 with an affected parent and sibling. Early feeding difficulties are common due to the difficulty in creating a negative intra-oral pressure for sucking, but are not universal. Orthodontic plates may be helpful, and breast feeding may be more successful. Long-term follow-up of speech and hearing is important.

3.  **BCE**
    The tongue in this syndrome is not large, but is posteriorly positioned (glossoptosis) and therefore tends to obstruct the airway. Airway obstruction is particularly severe in the supine position and therefore feeding problems are common. Recurrent airway obstruction may lead to pulmonary hypertension. Chromosomal abnormality is usually not present.

4.  **BCDE**
    Resistance to candida infection depends on normal cellular immunity. Candidiasis is common in a rare condition – DiGeorge syndrome – where there is absence of the thymus and therefore of T-lymphocytes. In normal babies antibiotics which suppress the normal mouth bacterial flora, and poor hygienic standards, inadequate sterilising of feeding bottles and teats and use of dummies, are all common factors causing recurrent oral thrush infection.

5. **Causes of oral ulceration in childhood include:**
   A. Stevens–Johnson syndrome.
   B. primary herpetic infection.
   C. chickenpox infection.
   D. coeliac disease.
   E. measles.

6. **Macroglossia is a feature of:**
   A. Down syndrome.
   B. hyperthyroidism.
   C. Hurler syndrome – mucopolysaccharidosis type 1.
   D. Beckwith syndrome.
   E. classical cleft lip and palate syndrome.

7. **The following are pathological conditions of the tongue which require treatment:**
   A. fissured or scrotal tongue.
   B. strawberry tongue.
   C. tongue tie.
   D. geographical tongue.
   E. median rhomboid glossitis.

8. **Teething is a recognised cause of:**
   A. febrile convulsions.
   B. diarrhoea.
   C. persistent pyrexia.
   D. irritability.
   E. haematemesis.

5. **ABC**
   Stevens–Johnson syndrome causes ulceration of the mouth with involvement of the conjunctivae and skin. There may be a number of triggers, including drugs (e.g. sulphonamides) or infections (e.g. mycoplasma). A child's primary Herpes simplex infection commonly presents as a herpetic stomatitis. Chickenpox commonly produces oral vesicles and ulceration. Measles produces koplik spots over the buccal mucosa but without ulceration. Crohn's disease but not coeliac disease may cause oral ulceration.

6. **ACD**
   Enlargement of the tongue occurs in hy*po*thyroidism. Beckwith syndrome is a condition characterised by generalised viscero-megaly at birth as a result of hyperinsulinism in utero. The major life-threatening complication of this condition is severe neonatal hypoglycaemia. In common cleft lip and palate syndrome there is no enlargement of the tongue.

7. **B**
   Fissured tongue is found as a congenital and sometimes familial abnormality in a small number of healthy individuals and fairly commonly in Down syndrome. In geographical tongue there are a number of smooth red areas on the tongue with greyish margins. These areas change shape and position as the filiform papillae desquamate and regenerate. Median rhomboid glossi-tis represents a midline, smooth oval patch of congenitally absent papillae – there are no symptoms. Tongue tie – i.e. ankyloglossia – is a common condition. The lingual frenulum normally extends almost to the tip of the tongue in infants and recedes during childhood. Treatment is very rarely required. Strawberry tongue may be found in a variety of conditions such as Streptococcal infections and Kawasaki disease.

8. **D**
   The medically correct answer to this question is that teething produces only teeth, maybe with a little discomfort and irritability. Many parents and grandparents would disagree, ascribing a whole host of symptoms to the expected appearance of teeth.

9. **Delayed teething is associated with:**
   A. rickets.
   B. fragile X syndrome of mental retardation.
   C. hypothyroidism.
   D. breast feeding.
   E. Down syndrome.

10. **Discolouration of the teeth may be found after:**
   A. prolonged neonatal hyperbilirubinaemia.
   B. administration of iron supplements.
   C. prolonged phenytoin administration.
   D. administration of fluoride supplements.
   E. treatment of respiratory infections in infancy with tetracycline.

11. **The following may cause a fluctuant swelling** *in the neck:*
   A. cystic hygroma.
   B. bronchogenic cyst.
   C. branchial cyst.
   D. thyroglossal cyst.
   E. tuberculous lymphadenitis.

12. **The following may cause swelling of the side of the face and cheek:**
   A. mumps.
   B. infectious mononucleosis.
   C. Staphylococcal parotitis.
   D. lymphoma of the parotid.
   E. measles.

9. **ACE**

The primary teeth begin to erupt between 6 months (incisors) and 2 years (second molars). The timing of eruption of the teeth depends on skeletal maturity, which may be delayed in the conditions indicated above. Method of feeding does not affect the timing of teething. Delayed teething is not a marker for mental retardation, though some mentally retarded children may have delayed teething – i.e. children with Down syndrome.

10. **ABDE**

Prolonged jaundice may permanently stain teeth green/yellow. Oral iron may cause temporary grey staining of teeth. Tetracycline administered during development of the primary or secondary dentition (up to 7 years of age) may cause permanent staining of the teeth. Excessive fluoride supplementation will produce an irregular mottling of the teeth. Phenytoin may cause gingival hyperplasia but does not affect the development of the teeth themselves.

11. **ACDE**

Cystic hygroma is a lymphatic abnormality which classically occurs in the neck and may extend retrosternally. Bronchogenic cysts are intrathoracic. Branchial cysts typically present as a swelling or sinus anterior to the sternomastoid muscle. Thyroglossal cysts may be found anywhere along the course of the thyroglossal duct from the tongue to the thyroid isthmus. A caseating TB gland may present as a fluctuating cervical abscess.

12. **ABCD**

Inflammation and swelling of the parotid is characteristic of mumps infection and can rarely occur after MMR vaccination. Suppurative parotitis can occur and *S. aureus* is commonly the causative organism. Lymphoma may involve the parotid or the pre-auricular nodes, which would then enlarge as they would also in glandular fever (EB virus infection). Measles may cause redness of the face with circumoral pallor but usually not significant swelling of the face.

13. **The diagnosis of an H-type tracheo-oesophageal fistula would be suggested by:**
    A. polyhydramnios in pregnancy.
    B. difficulty in swallowing secretions after birth.
    C. failure successfully to pass a nasogastric tube.
    D. recurrent chest infections.
    E. persistent abdominal distension.

14. **Immediate treatment of a baby with suspected oesophageal atresia should consist of:**
    A. continuous aspiration of the upper oesophageal pouch.
    B. passage of a nasogastric tube for feeding.
    C. intravenous fluid infusion.
    D. intubation and ventilation.
    E. urgent transfer to a surgical neonatal surgical unit.

15. **After repair of a tracheo-oesphageal atresia and fistula, the following immediate and longer-term complications should be anticipated:**
    A. difficulty in swallowing lumpy food.
    B. inability to cough.
    C. pneumothorax.
    D. reflux oesophagitis.
    E. empyema.

16. **A child who has swallowed an unknown quantity of a strong solution of bleach should:**
    A. be allowed home if there is no ulceration of the lips or tongue.
    B. have vomiting induced with ipecac.
    C. be investigated with a barium swallow.
    D. be investigated by an early endoscopy.
    E. be offered copious drinks of milk.

**13.  DE**

A, B and C are all suggestive of oesophageal *atresia*. Isolated tracheo-oesophageal fistula (TOF) without atresia occurs in only 4% of TOFs. As a result of aspiration of stomach contents through the fistula into the airway, presentation is with recurrent episodes of pneumonia – commonly affecting the right upper lobe. If air is forced through the fistula with crying, then gaseous abdominal distension results.

**14.  ACE**

Saliva must be continuously aspirated from the oesophageal pouch to prevent aspiration into the lungs. A nasogastric tube cannot be passed as there is oesophageal atresia. Intravenous fluids are necessary to replace the baby's fluid and electrolyte losses and to maintain the blood sugar. Unless the baby has respiratory difficulty, there is no need for elective ventilation. The baby should be transferred to a neonatal surgical unit because there is usually a fistula from the lower oesophageal pouch to the trachea which must be identified and closed as soon as possible.

**15.  ACDE**

Acute complications of an anastomosis leak include pneumothorax, mediastinitis or empyema. A contrast swallow is carried out before feeding is started. Anastomotic stricture is not uncommon and is more likely if the oesophageal anastomosis was sutured under tension. A stricture causes difficulty in swallowing and may require repeated oesophageal dilatation. Gastro-oesophageal reflux is common and may be associated with a hiatus hernia. These babies often have a loud, rattling cough ('TOF cough') which is caused by difficulty in clearing secretions past a segment of tracheomalacia at the site of the (closed) tracheal fistula.

**16.  DE**

All children who have ingested caustic fluid should be admitted. The presence or absence of oropharyngeal lesions is no guide to the presence or severity of oesophageal damage. Vomiting should not be induced as this risks aspiration of damaging fluids into the lungs. Early endoscopy within the first 24 hours is the best way to assess oesophageal ulceration. Immediate first-aid treatment following caustic ingestion includes the encouragement of milk drinks.

17. **Causes of vomiting and failure to thrive** *at 4 months* **of age include:**
    A. pyloric stenosis.
    B. gastro-oesophageal reflux.
    C. coeliac disease.
    D. duodenal atresia.
    E. urinary tract infection.

18. **An exclusively breast-fed baby girl of 6 months suffers a haematemesis – possible diagnoses include:**
    A. oesophagitis.
    B. vitamin K deficiency.
    C. haemophilia A.
    D. duodenal ulcer.
    E. oesophageal varices due to portal hypertension.

19. **The classical findings in infantile hypertrophic pyloric stenosis include:**
    A. effortless vomiting.
    B. visible gastric peristalsis.
    C. a palpable, hypertrophied pylorus.
    D. a metabolic acidosis.
    E. hyperchloraemia.

20. **Infantile hypertrophic pyloric stenosis:**
    A. is commoner in girls than boys.
    B. commonly presents with poor feeding.
    C. should be treated as a surgical emergency.
    D. is associated with an unconjugated hyperbilirubinaemia.
    E. can be diagnosed reliably by ultrasound scanning.

17.  **BE**

     Pyloric stenosis occurs between 3 weeks and 3 months of age.
     Gastro-oesophageal reflux is a common cause of vomiting but
     most affected babies thrive. Coeliac disease is unlikely as solids
     should not be started before 4 months of age. Duodenal atresia
     presents with early-onset vomiting in the neonatal period.
     Chronic infection of the urinary tract, particularly if associated
     with an obstructive lesion, may be an underlying cause of
     vomiting and poor weight gain.

18.  **ABDE**

     Haemophilia will not cause symptoms of bleeding *in girls*.
     Oesophagitis may result in haematemesis, usually after reflux
     and recurrent vomiting. Vitamin K deficiency may occur in
     exclusively breast-fed infants and may present with late-onset
     haemorrhagic disease – formula milk is protective. Infantile
     portal hypertension with varices may result from neonatal
     umbilical vein catheterisation or umbilical sepsis causing portal
     vein thrombosis. Splenomegaly should always be present if
     there is significant portal hypertension. Peptic ulceration may
     occur at any age.

19.  **BC**

     In pyloric stenosis vomiting is usually forceful. Gastric peristalsis
     spreads from the left hypochondrium towards the right iliac
     fossa. The hypertrophied pylorus may be felt lateral to the *right*
     rectus muscle. If the stomach is very distended, the pylorus may
     be palpated more easily immediately after the baby has vomited.
     Repeated vomiting of gastric acid causes a metabolic alkalosis
     and hy*po*chloraemia. Aldosterone secretion results in prefer-
     ential reabsorption of $Na^+$ at the distal tubule and therefore loss
     of $K^+$ and $H^+$ ions – thus the urine is paradoxically acidic despite
     the plasma alkalosis.

20.  **DE**

     Pyloric stenosis is commoner in boys than girls; the ratio is 4:1.
     The babies are ready to feed again soon after vomiting. The
     condition must be *medically* stabilised and the fluid, electrolyte
     and metabolic alkalosis corrected with intravenous saline and
     potassium before surgery. There is increased efficiency of the
     enterohepatic circulation of bile in high intestinal obstruction
     causing clinical jaundice. Ultrasound reliably demonstrates the
     elongated and hypertrophied pylorus.

21. **Congenital duodenal obstruction is associated with:**
    A. polyhydramnios in pregnancy.
    B. bile-stained vomiting.
    C. Turner syndrome.
    D. congenital malformation of the pancreas.
    E. marked abdominal distension.

22. **Regarding the digestion of carbohydrate:**
    A. carbohydrate digestion begins in the mouth.
    B. amylase is a brush border enzyme.
    C. glucose and galactose are digested by brush border disaccharidase enzyme.
    D. all sugars are absorbed by an active transport process.
    E. maltose, maltotriose and amylopectin are breakdown products of starch.

23. **Regarding the digestion of protein:**
    A. protein digestion begins in the mouth.
    B. protein is digested in the small bowel by brush border enzymes.
    C. amino acids are absorbed by passive diffusion.
    D. mucosal enterokinase causes release of pancreatic proteolytic enzymes.
    E. proteins may be absorbed intact across the gut mucosa.

24. **The following are necessary for normal fat absorption:**
    A. normal small bowel villus architecture.
    B. normal brush border enzymes.
    C. normal endocrine pancreatic function.
    D. bilirubin.
    E. micelle formation.

21. **ABD**

Upper GI obstruction or failure of normal swallowing will lead to increasing polyhydramnios over the last trimester of pregnancy. A detailed antenatal ultrasound scan may show the stomach and first part of duodenum distended with fluid. After delivery, the classical, 'double bubble', appearance may be seen on abdominal X-ray, once the upper GI tract has become filled with air. As the obstruction is usually distal to the ampulla of Vater, bilious vomiting is common. Duodenal atresia is associated with Down syndrome. There is an annular pancreas encircling the duodenum in 30%. Distension does not occur as the distal bowel is airless.

22. **AE**

Starch digestion begins with salivary amylase in the mouth. Pancreatic amylase continues that process. Starch is broken down into amylose – a glucose polymer – and then to maltose and maltotriose (glucose doublets and triplets). Monosaccharides glucose and galactose are actively absorbed by an energy-dependent pump process, fructose and xylose by facilitated diffusion. Disaccharides lactose, maltose, sucrose and amylopectin are digested by the brush border enzymes before absorption as monosaccharides.

23. **DE**

Protein digestion begins in the stomach under the action of acid and pepsin. Proteolytic enzymes are released from the pancreas after stimulation by enterokinase. Proteases reduce protein to amino acids and oligopeptides. Oligopeptides may be absorbed and hydrolysed by intracellular peptidases. Amino acids are absorbed by specific active transport systems. Occasionally whole proteins may be absorbed intact – this is more likely to happen in the neonatal gut.

24. **AE**

Fat absorption is dependent on emulsification of fat in the stomach. Bile salts are required for lipase (from the exocrine pancreas) to break down fat into monoglycerides (MGs) and fatty acids (FAs). Micelles are formed and the MGs and FAs pass into the mucosal cell, are then re-esterified and form chylomicrons. Short and medium chain triglycerides do not need to be broken down prior to absorption, but are taken up directly from the bowel into the mucosal cell.

25. **The following investigations will confirm the presence of malabsorption:**
    A. a sweat test.
    B. 3-day faecal fat estimation.
    C. xylose absorption test.
    D. upper GI endoscopy.
    E. antigliadin antibody test.

26. **Features of a large bowel intestinal obstruction include:**
    A. constipation.
    B. abdominal distension.
    C. absence of bowel sounds.
    D. early onset of vomiting.
    E. lower abdominal pain.

27. **Typical features of ileocolic intussusception include:**
    A. greatest incidence in the first 2 years of life.
    B. symptoms of painless intestinal obstruction.
    C. passage of blood in the stool.
    D. an increased risk associated with any bowel wall abnormality.
    E. a palpable abdominal mass.

28. **Lactose malabsorption would be suggested by:**
    A. increased breath hydrogen.
    B. watery stools.
    C. alkaline stools on pH testing.
    D. abdominal distension.
    E. a positive clinitest reaction on testing the faecal fluid.

25. **BC**

The sweat test will usually establish a diagnosis of cystic fibrosis but not all CF patients have malabsorption. Similarly, not all patients with a positive antigliadin antibody test will have coeliac disease. Upper GI endoscopy will not establish a diagnosis of malabsorption. Faecal fat excretion should be less than 10% of fat intake and values greater than 5 g/day would indicate fat malabsorption. Xylose absorption is a rather old-fashioned test of jejunal mucosal function.

26. **ABE**

Classical large bowel obstructive symptoms include delayed vomiting, absolute constipation, distension and colicky lower abdominal pain. Bowel sounds are periodically increased, associated with waves of peristalsis. Vomiting occurs early in high intestinal obstruction and late in low intestinal obstruction.

27. **ACDE**

Intussusception is commonest in children under 2 years. The condition may present after an intercurrent infection. The commonest presenting symptom is intermittent, severe colicky abdominal pain, causing intermittent inconsolable screaming. Young infants may demonstrate intense vagal effects with shock, hypotension, shallow breathing or even apnoea. Vomiting is common and may provide some temporary relief. When the bowel becomes oedematous and ischaemic, rectal bleeding may occur ('redcurrant jelly stools'), but this is usually a late sign. The abdominal mass may be difficult to feel unless examined between episodes of pain. Any bowel wall abnormality may act as the lead point of the intussusceptum – i.e. bowel wall lymphoid tissue, a polyp or an adherent faecal mass as in cystic fibrosis.

28. **ABDE**

Undigested lactose retains water within the bowel and is fermented by large bowel bacteria producing organic acids and gas. Hydrogen from sugar fermentation is present in increased concentration in the expired air. Abdominal distension is often present. The explosive, watery and *acid* stool produces marked excoriation of the skin of the perianal region. Lactose is a reducing sugar and may produce a positive clinitest reaction – this is not a totally reliable test. Pain is not a major feature.

**29. Lactose intolerance may occur:**
- **A.** as a congenital abnormality.
- **B.** in extreme preterm infants as a result of GI tract immaturity.
- **C.** following gastroenteritis.
- **D.** in coeliac disease.
- **E.** as a result of pancreatic insufficiency.

**30. Jejunal villus atrophy is associated with:**
- **A.** cystic fibrosis.
- **B.** Hirschsprung's disease.
- **C.** cow's milk protein intolerance.
- **D.** Crohn's disease.
- **E.** gluten sensitivity.

**31. Coeliac disease is associated with:**
- **A.** HLA-B8 antigen.
- **B.** dermatitis herpetiformis.
- **C.** temporary sensitivity to gluten.
- **D.** increased risk of bowel lymphoma.
- **E.** delayed puberty.

**32. Coeliac disease is characterised by:**
- **A.** involvement of the whole of the small bowel.
- **B.** increased numbers of plasma cells in the lamina propria.
- **C.** atrophy of the crypts of Lieberkühn.
- **D.** increased numbers of intra-epithelial lymphocytes.
- **E.** proximal jejunal villus atrophy.

**29. ABCD**

Lactose intolerance may rarely result from congenital lactase deficiency. Much more commonly this is an acquired defect. This may occur when there has been damage to the brush border enzymes of the small intestinal villi, as commonly happens transiently after gastroenteritis, in other upper GI infections such as giardiasis or when the villi themselves are abnormal as in coeliac disease and other conditions causing villus atrophy.

**30. CE**

Villus atrophy is not a feature of cystic fibrosis, Hirschsprung's disease or Crohn's disease. Cow's milk protein intolerance and coeliac disease are well-recognised causes of partial or total villus atrophy.

**31. ABDE**

HLA-B8 individuals have a tenfold increase in risk of developing coeliac disease. HLA-B8 incidence is higher in the Irish population than any other in Europe. Dermatitis herpetiformis – an itchy skin eruption – is uncommon in children, but it is usually associated with villus atrophy which responds to a gluten-free diet. Except for a few very young children who may develop a transient gluten intolerance, coeliac disease is a lifelong condition. Abandonment of the gluten-free diet in adult life may not provoke symptoms, but significantly increases the risk of bowel lymphoma. Teenagers with undiagnosed coeliac disease may be asymptomatic apart from delayed onset of puberty.

**32. BDE**

The proximal small bowel is most involved in coeliac disease. The distal small bowel is usually normal. This is in keeping with the theory that it is the gluten which is toxic to the bowel, and that hydrolysed gluten is harmless. It has been shown that gluten instilled into the distal small bowel induces the typical mucosal changes. The typical biopsy changes are of villus atrophy, lengthening of the crypts, a plasma cell infiltrate of the lamina propria and increased numbers of intra-epithelial lymphocytes (CD8 cells). This latter abnormality may be the only finding in some children with mild or early changes.

33. **The following conditions are associated with malabsorption:**
    A. cystic fibrosis.
    B. intestinal giardiasis.
    C. gastro-oesophageal reflux.
    D. ulcerative colitis.
    E. pyloric stenosis.

34. **The following are features of Crohn's disease:**
    A. full-thickness bowel wall involvement.
    B. continuous involvement of the large bowel.
    C. bloody diarrhoea.
    D. granuloma formation.
    E. perianal abscess formation.

35. **The following are associated with Crohn's disease:**
    A. onycholysis.
    B. cataracts.
    C. arthritis.
    D. precocious puberty.
    E. bile salt deficiency.

36. **In ulcerative colitis the typical pathological findings include:**
    A. mucosal ulceration of the rectum which extends a variable distance proximally.
    B. giant cell granuloma formation.
    C. true polyp formation.
    D. stricture formation.
    E. chronic hepatitis in 10%.

**33.   AB**
Pancreatic malabsorption occurs in cystic fibrosis, and carbohydrate malabsorption may occur following acute gastroenteritis as a result of disaccharidase enzyme loss from the brush
border. Gastro-oesophageal reflux and pyloric stenosis are not
associated with malabsorption. Crohn's disease affecting the
small bowel (not ulcerative colitis) is associated with malabsorption.

**34.   ACDE**
Crohn's disease causes inflammation of the full thickness of the
bowel wall. Any part of the bowel from mouth to anus may be
affected. Discontinuous lesions are typical, the so-called 'skip
lesions'. Granuloma formation is characteristic of Crohn's
disease but may not always be present. Perianal abscesses or
fistulae may occur. Abdominal pain is the characteristic
symptom of Crohn's disease. Bloody *diarrhoea* is more typical
of ulcerative colitis but may occur in all inflammatory bowel
disease.

**35.   CE**
Onycholysis – i.e. separation of the fingernails from the nail bed
– occurs in psoriasis. Finger clubbing may occur in inflammatory bowel disease. Cataracts do not occur, except as a possible
very late effect of chronic uveitis or long-term steroid therapy.
Uveitis presents as a sore, gritty, red eye with reduced visual
acuity. Other possible systemic manifestations include arthritis
and erythema nodosum. Bile salt deficiency may occur if the
terminal ileum is affected and thus the enterohepatic circulation of bile inhibited. Delayed puberty is common in Crohn's
disease.

**36.   AE**
Ulcerative colitis (UC) affects the mucosa and submucosa and
extends a variable distance proximally. Granuloma and stricture
formation are more typical of Crohn's disease than ulcerative
colitis. Pseudopolyps are a feature of colitis when irregular
longitudinal ulcers leave isolated islands of oedematous
mucosa. A chronic active or even a suppurative hepatitis with
micro abscesses (suppurative pyelitis) may occur.

37. **The following statements are *more true* of Crohn's disease than ulcerative colitis (UC):**
    A. fistula formation is common.
    B. a featureless bowel with loss of haustration is seen on barium enema.
    C. toxic dilatation of the colon is a potentially fatal complication.
    D. there is an increased risk of malignancy.
    E. relapses may be prevented by long-term sulphasalazine.

38. **Hirschsprung's disease:**
    A. affects both sexes equally.
    B. may affect any part of the bowel.
    C. has an increased incidence in Down syndrome.
    D. always presents in the neonatal period.
    E. is usually associated with a distended rectum loaded with faeces.

39. **Delayed passage of meconium in the newborn period is a common feature of:**
    A. duodenal atresia.
    B. anal atresia.
    C. cystic fibrosis.
    D. Hirschsprung's disease.
    E. breast-fed infants.

40. **Colitis is associated with:**
    A. cow's milk protein allergy.
    B. coeliac disease.
    C. giardia infection.
    D. Campylobacter infection.
    E. Hirschsprung's disease.

**37.  A**

Strictures and fistulas are more typical of Crohn's disease than UC. All the rest are more common in UC. Toxic dilatation is an important complication presenting with fever, abdominal distension and pain. There is circulatory compromise leading on to collapse and/or perforation. Sulphasalazine and 5-aminosalicylates are used in both UC and Crohn's disease but have greater effectiveness in the former.

**38.  C**

Overall, males are more commonly affected than females. The condition may affect a variable amount of the bowel from the rectum extending proximally. The extent of the disease – and the level of resection – is usually assessed by serial biopsies. While the condition usually presents in the neonatal period, presentation later in infancy or childhood with chronic constipation is not uncommon. There is an association with Down syndrome. The rectum is usually narrow and empty on rectal examination.

**39.  BCD**

Babies with anal atresia are unable to pass meconium, for obvious reasons. Duodenal atresia will prevent food passing beyond the foregut, so there will be a delay in passing changing stools, though meconium may be passed normally at first. Breast-fed babies should pass meconium normally. Meconium ileus, due to sticky meconium and an associated microcolon, may occur in cystic fibrosis – the microcolon does not cause problems once the abnormal meconium has been evacuated. Hirschsprung's disease commonly presents as neonatal bowel obstruction.

**40.  ADE**

Any of the organisms causing dysentery-like syndromes, such as Campylobacter, *E. coli*, Shigella or Salmonella, may cause an infective colitis. *Giardia lamblia* is a protozoal parasite, which may be chronically carried in the small bowel, and may cause symptoms of malabsorption, but does not cause colitis. Food allergy may cause an allergic colitis recognisable histologically by an eosinophilic infiltrate in the submucosa. Hirschsprung's disease is associated with an enterocolitis, a severe inflammatory process involving the bowel wall, which may lead to perforation and peritonitis. Coeliac disease affects only the proximal small bowel.

41. **Causes of constipation in childhood include:**
    A. coercive potty training.
    B. acute febrile illness.
    C. a change of diet.
    D. abnormal family dynamics.
    E. painful defecation.

42. **Children suffering from constipation with overflow have:**
    A. low self-esteem.
    B. long-term psychological disorders.
    C. an acquired megacolon/megarectum.
    D. a history of regular faecal smearing.
    E. daytime soiling only.

43. **Constipation in a 5-year-old is more likely to be due to a significant primary cause than to simple constipation if associated with:**
    A. colicky abdominal pain.
    B. abdominal distension.
    C. reflex anal dilatation.
    D. a height velocity on the 3rd centile.
    E. secondary diurnal enuresis.

44. **The mother of 6-week-old fully breast-fed baby reports to you that for the past month her baby has been crying inconsolably. Crying occurs every day, especially during the evening when the crying often lasts for up to 3 hours at a time. In between bouts of crying the baby appears well. Loose seedy stools are passed on alternate days. The baby's height and weight are increasing along the 75th centile and there is nothing abnormal to find on thorough physical examination. You should:**
    A. admit the child to hospital as an emergency.
    B. change the baby on to formula milk feeds.
    C. carry out a rectal examination in case the child has constipation.
    D. arrange an abdominal ultrasound scan to exclude intussusception.
    E. reassure the mother and monitor the baby's progress.

**41. ABCDE**

All of these are correct – B and C frequently lead to the passage of a hard stool that may cause pain resulting in a reluctance to defecate. The child 'holds on', leading to distension of the rectum, loss of normal sensation of rectal fullness and constipation with overflow. Abnormal potty training routines in toddlers or disturbed family relationships in older children may be associated with constipation.

**42. AC**

Constipation with overflow is an acquired condition and is commonly associated with an acquired megacolon or rectum. Although often associated with a low self-esteem, constipation is not usually associated with major psychological disturbance. Regular smearing of faeces on walls or furniture or hiding soiled underclothes is more typical of encopresis and psychological disturbance than 'simple' constipation with overflow. Faecal soiling in constipated children may occur day or night.

**43. DE**

Constipation is commonly associated with colicky abdominal pain and abdominal distension when there is significant loading of the bowel. Reflex anal dilatation was (in)famously and erroneously used as a diagnostic test of anal sexual abuse. With the child lying in the lateral position, the buttocks are gently parted and the anus may dilate. Anal dilatation may be a normal finding and is sometimes seen in constipated children. A height *velocity* on the 3rd centile is always abnormal and, together with constipation, is suggestive of hypothyroidism. Secondary diurnal enuresis and constipation in a 5-year-old suggests an emotional or physical problem needing careful evaluation.

**44. E**

This is a classic history of '3-month colic'. Offering admission to hospital, if the mother is reaching the end of her tether, is appropriate but this is not a medical emergency. As the baby is well and thriving, there is no need for any investigation. Antispasmodic drugs may be of some benefit. It would be wrong to stop the baby breast feeding unless there was reason to suspect allergy to cow's milk protein. Infrequent soft stools are common in some breast-fed babies. Reassurance and explanation are usually all that is needed.

**45. Constipation is common in:**
   A. hypothyroidism.
   B. lead poisoning.
   C. Hirschsprung's disease.
   D. Down syndrome.
   E. hypercalcaemia.

**45. ABCDE – all of these**
Idiopathic hypercalcaemia is rare, but it is associated with abdominal pain, vomiting and constipation. Lead poisoning is now uncommon in the UK and is associated with a hypochromic anaemia, basophilic stippling of the red cells, constipation, abdominal pain, vomiting and, more seriously, mental changes and encephalopathy. In short-segment Hirschsprung's disease presentation may occur outside the neonatal period with abdominal distension and constipation.

# 14

# Genetics

1. **Regarding Down syndrome:**
   A. the incidence is 1 in 1500.
   B. the palpebral fissures slope upwards.
   C. Brushfield spots are found in the mouth.
   D. microglossia causes speech delay.
   E. a single palmar crease is pathognomonic of the syndrome.

2. **The child with Down syndrome:**
   A. has a 10–20 times higher risk of leukaemia than the normal population.
   B. has a 40–60% chance of congenital heart disease.
   C. will have an IQ from 20 to 75.
   D. will be infertile if male.
   E. is more likely to have an elderly mother.

3. **Regarding patients with fragile X syndrome:**
   A. the incidence is 1 in 1000.
   B. females are more severely affected than males.
   C. they have hypogonadotrophic hypogonadism.
   D. the diagnosis is best made by demonstrating folate-sensitive fragile site on chromosome analysis.
   E. 50% are blind secondary to optic atrophy.

4. **The following genetic disorders are inherited as X-linked recessive:**
   A. Haemophilia A.
   B. achondroplasia.
   C. myotonic dystrophy.
   D. congenital spherocytosis.
   E. cystic fibrosis.

1. **B**

   The incidence of Down syndrome is 1 in 700 live births. The clinical diagnosis is made by a constellation of features none of which are pathognomonic of the syndrome and include: upward sloping palpebral fissures – i.e. the outer canthus is higher than the inner; and Brushfield spots – white speckling of the iris. The tongue appears large and may protrude as the mouth is small.

2. **ABCD**

   Males are infertile; however, females are fertile. They are at increased risk of congenital heart disease, particularly atrioventricular canal defects. They have a 10–20 times increased risk of developing leukaemia. They have a low IQ. Early developmental milestones are eventually reached and the earlier assessment of development tends to be more favourable than the formal measurement of IQ in later childhood. The risk increases with the age of the mother; the incidence for mothers aged 25 is 1 in 1400 and increases to 1 in 46 for mothers aged 45. However most babies with Down Syndrome will be born to young mothers.

3. **A**

   Fragile X syndrome was initially diagnosed by detecting folate-sensitive fragile sites. The diagnosis now is made by detection of DNA repeats at Xq27 locus. The incidence is 1 in 1000. Males are more severely affected than females, and it is now recognised as the second commonest cause of mental handicap in males after Down syndrome. They have typical facial features with a large forehead, large head, long nose, prominent chin and long ears. Macro-orchidism is present in 80% of adult fragile X males and 15% of prepubertal boys – the large testes are functionally normal. They do not have optic atrophy.

4. **A**

   Haemophilia A and B are inherited as X-linked recessive. Achondroplasia is inherited as autosomal dominant, or occurs as a spontaneous mutation in up to one-third of cases. Myotonic dystrophy is inherited as autosomal dominant – the clinical phenotype varies according to whether the abnormal chromosome is maternal or paternal. Congenital spherocytosis is inherited as autosomal dominant. Cystic fibrosis is inherited as autosomal recessive.

5. **The following genetic disorders can reliably be detected antenatally by chorionic villus sampling:**
   A. Down syndrome.
   B. fragile X.
   C. spina bifida.
   D. Pierre Robin syndrome.
   E. congenital adrenal hyperplasia.

6. **The following are definitions of descriptive terms used in dysmorphology:**
   A. *clinodactyly* means small hands.
   B. *hypertelorism* means increased distance between the ears.
   C. *brachycephaly* means flat forehead.
   D. *phocomelia* means absence of limb.
   E. *philtrum* means vertical folds on upper lip.

7. **Regarding Turner syndrome:**
   A. the incidence is 1 in 3000.
   B. the karyotype is 45XO in 60% of cases.
   C. there is an increased incidence of Turner syndrome for the mother's future pregnancies.
   D. mental retardation is typical with an IQ of 50–75.
   E. diagnosis is typically made by fibroblast culture.

8. **The diagnosis of Turner syndrome should be suspected if:**
   A. a baby has lymphoedema of the hands and feet.
   B. a girl presents with precocious puberty.
   C. the carrying angle at the elbow is increased.
   D. there is evidence of hemihypertrophy.
   E. a child has pulmonary stenosis.

5. **AE**

Chorionic villus sampling is used to detect some genetic disorders at 10–12 weeks' gestation. Down syndrome is reliably detected by this method. The fragile X site is not reliably expressed in chorionic villus material or amniocytes, so the prenatal diagnosis depends on fetal blood sampling. Spina bifida is detected on detailed ultrasound scanning. Pierre Robin occurs sporadically and the exact genetic problem is not known. Congenital adrenal hyperplasia can be detected but an index case is required to initiate the process of antenatal detection.

6. **DE**

*Clinodactyly* means incurving, usually of the 5th digit. *Hypertelorism* means increased distance between the eyes. *Brachycephaly* means flat occiput. *Phocomelia* means absence; *rhizomelia* proximal segment shortening; *mesomelia* middle segment shortening; and *acromelia* distal segment shortening of a limb.

7. **AB**

The incidence of Turner syndrome at birth is 1 in 3000, though it is a frequent finding in first trimester abortions. The classic karyotype, 45XO, is present in about 60% of girls with the syndrome. Other sex chromosome abnormalities may be associated with the syndrome, including mosaicism, ring chromosomes and deletions. There is no increased risk of recurrence in further pregnancies. Girls with Turner syndrome are of normal IQ, although they may have specific learning difficulties, especially in spatial perception. The diagnosis is made by culture of peripheral lymphocytes – in mosaics the culture of skin fibroblasts may be helpful.

8. **AC**

At birth a girl with Turner syndrome may have lymphoedema of the hands and feet. The webbing of the neck present in some girls results from lymphoedema of the neck in utero. Other typical features include a wide carrying angle at the elbow; widely spaced nipples with a shield-shaped chest; cardiac abnormalities, typically coarctation of the aorta; clinodactyly; abnormal nails; and renal tract anomalies. They may present with short stature and delayed puberty. Ovarian failure is typical with streak ovaries.

9. **Regarding Klinefelter syndrome:**
   A. the incidence is 1 in 1000.
   B. the testes are small and atrophic.
   C. gynaecomastia indicates excess testosterone production.
   D. presentation is with short stature.
   E. there is an increased risk of breast cancer compared with normal males.

10. **Increased chromosome fragility is associated with the following:**
    A. Turner syndrome.
    B. congenital heart disease.
    C. ataxia telangiectasia.
    D. Down syndrome.
    E. cystic fibrosis.

9.  **ABE**

    The incidence of Klinefelter syndrome is 1 in 1000. The usual presentation is with tall stature, with disproportionately long legs and small testes for apparent degree of virilisation or infertility. The testes are small and there is poor testosterone production, which is inadequate to fuse the epiphyses at the appropriate time. There is often marked pubertal gynaecomastia and the risk of breast malignancy is the same as for females.

10. **CD**

    Increased chromosome fragility is a recognised feature of some disorders and may predispose to malignancy. Ataxia telangiectasia is characterised by progressive neurological deterioration and telangiectasia of conjunctivae and skin. There is a high incidence of malignant disease and immunodeficiency, related to the DNA repair defect. Down syndrome is also associated with increased fragility and these children have an increased risk of malignancy, particularly ALL.

# 15

## Feeding and Nutrition

1. **In breast milk:**
   A. the main carbohydrate source is glucose.
   B. the colostrum is rich in fats.
   C. the majority of protein is easily digestible whey.
   D. the majority of energy is derived from carbohydrate.
   E. there is a higher fat content in cold weather.

2. **The benefits of breast milk compared to modified cow's milk are:**
   A. increased caloric value.
   B. increased protection from HIV infection in HIV-positive mothers.
   C. increased calcium content.
   D. decreased risk of gastroenteritis in developed countries.
   E. decreased risk of haemorrhagic disease of newborn.

3. **Regarding infant feeding and growth:**
   A. the fluid intake should be a minimum of 200 ml/kg/24 hours.
   B. average weight gain should be 200 g/week.
   C. occipitofrontal circumference should double from birth to 1 year.
   D. birth weight should double by 6 months.
   E. average energy intake required for normal growth is 100 kcal/kg/24 hours.

4. **When weaning an infant (changing from purely milk feeds to a normal diet):**
   A. solids should not be introduced before 6 months of age.
   B. cow's milk should not be introduced before 18 months of age.
   C. the weaning diet will fully replace the milk diet by 1 year.
   D. foods such as eggs should be avoided.
   E. food should be liquidised until 18 months of age.

1. **CE**

   Breast milk is composed of protein, fat and carbohydrate with many additional elements. Colostrum is rich in protein, particularly immunoglobulins. Established breast milk carbohydrate is lactose – glucose and galactose. The protein is easily hydrolysed whey (lactalbumen). Fat provides the main calorie source. The human does adapt to colder conditions by increasing the breast milk fat content.

2. **D**

   There are many advantages to breast feeding. There is reduced risk of respiratory and GI infection even in developed countries. However, there is a risk of transmitting infection; in the developed countries women are advised not to breast-feed if HIV infected. In Third World countries, despite the risk of HIV transmission, it is still safer to breast-feed because of the very high mortality rate in bottle-fed babies. The calcium content of breast milk is not increased. The vitamin K content of breast milk is low, so to prevent haemorrhagic disease of the newborn all parents are advised of the need for vitamin K injection.

3. **BDE**

   The milk intake should be 100–150 ml/kg/24 hours and thus 70–100 kcal/kg/24 hours to enable average growth of 200 g/week and thereby doubling birthweight by 5–6 months and trebling by 1 year. Head growth is proportionately much slower and even by adulthood has not doubled in circumference.

4. **D**

   Weaning involves the gradual introduction of solid feeds and usually commences around 4 months. It is necessary to supplement the diet at times of increased energy and mineral requirements as breast milk alone does not have sufficient quantities of iron, zinc, protein and possibly calories after 6 months. The child continues to consume significant quantities of milk for many months. It is sensible not to expose the infant to high allergenic-potential foods such as eggs and nuts. Cow's milk can be introduced from 6 months, but introduction is better delayed until 1 year as breast milk and formula milk contain significant amounts of iron and vitamins.

5. **The child fed a vegan diet will be at an increased risk of:**
   A. iron deficiency.
   B. rickets.
   C. megaloblastic anaemia.
   D. dental caries.
   E. scurvy.

6. **In nutritional rickets:**
   A. the incidence is increased in Asians.
   B. failure of calcium absorption from gut results in decreased PTH secretion.
   C. plasma alkaline phosphatase will be low, reflecting poor bone growth.
   D. examination may show expansion of the anterior ends of the bony ribs.
   E. full antirachitic activity of vitamin D is dependent on normal adrenal function.

7. **Regarding obesity:**
   A. one-third of obese adults date the onset of obesity to their childhood.
   B. children with simple obesity are usually short.
   C. obesity is not commonly due to a pathological condition.
   D. Cushing's syndrome causes centripetal obesity.
   E. obesity is common in Prader–Willi syndrome.

8. **In protein-energy malnutrition**
   A. marasmus results from low protein and low carbohydrate intake.
   B. kwashiorkor is known as weanlings' disease.
   C. kwashiorkor results from a high carbohydrate, no protein diet.
   D. the infant with marasmus has very poor prognosis.
   E. the child with kwashiorkor is oedematous.

5. **BC**

Vegans eat no animal products, including dairy products. Their diet will include cereals and vegetables, which are adequate sources of most vitamins and minerals, including iron. Vitamin $B_{12}$ is present in meat, fish, cheese and eggs and deficiency causes megaloblastic anaemia. Vitamin D is found in milk, cheese and liver and thus the vegan is at an increased risk of deficiency, which may cause rickets. Vitamin C is found in fresh fruit – deficiency is not likely. The vegan is not at increased risk of dental caries.

6. **AD**

Asians who do not expose their skin to sunlight and whose diet may be deficient in vitamin D are at increased risk of developing rickets. Hypocalcaemia stimulates increased parathyroid hormone secretion which mobilises calcium from the bone, increasing osteoclastic activity and so raising alkaline phosphatase levels. Vitamin D requires hydroxylation by liver and kidney (not adrenals) to be fully active. The child with rickets may show expansion of the ends of the long bones and ribs. Expansion of the rib ends at the costochondral junction is known as the 'rachitic rosary'.

7. **ACDE**

Obese adults were often obese children. Children with simple obesity are usually tall – energy intake, in part, dictates the rate of growth in early childhood. However, the final growth potential is not altered. There is rarely a pathological cause for obesity, but suspicions should be raised in the short, fat child. Cushing's syndrome causes abnormal fat distribution with typical 'lemon on matchsticks' appearance. Children with Prader–Willi syndrome have an insatiable appetite.

8. **ABCE**

Protein-energy malnutrition is a massive problem worldwide. The marasmic child is very skinny – as a result of a small but relatively balanced diet. The marasmic infant once fed a better diet will do well. Kwashiorkor results from a diet which contains good amounts of carbohydrate but no protein. Kwashiorkor is seen when the child is weaned commonly after the arrival of the next baby. Breast milk was providing the only source of protein. These children are oedematous because of low plasma oncotic pressure.

**9. The child who is failing to thrive:**

    **A.** is detected by the height and weight being greater than 3 standard deviations away from the mean.

    **B.** usually has an underlying medical condition.

    **C.** should be admitted to hospital and observed.

    **D.** should have faecal fat estimation to exclude malabsorption.

    **E.** needs careful dietary assessment.

**9.    E**

Diagnosis of failure to thrive cannot be made on a single measurement, however far from the mean. It is rather when the rate of growth fails to meet expected potential. There are a very large number of reasons, both medical and psychological, for failure to thrive. Usually there is no underlying pathological condition. Diagnosis depends on taking a detailed history – including dietary – and performing a detailed examination. The child rarely needs to undergo hospitalisation – all initial investigation should be performed on an outpatient basis. Faecal fat collection has little diagnostic value and is unpleasant to do! If malabsorption is suspected, a sweat test and a blood test for antigliadin antibodies (test for coeliac disease) should be performed. Inadequate intake is the commonest cause of poor weight gain because the child refuses to eat more, or less commonly because the child is deliberately starved.

# Minitest 4

1. **Bacterial endocarditis may occur in the following conditions:**
   A. hydrocephalus treated by ventriculo-peritoneal shunt.
   B. aortic stenosis.
   C. atrial septal defect.
   D. pulmonary stenosis.
   E. tetralogy of Fallot.

2. **Clinical findings in tuberose sclerosis include:**
   A. depigmented macules over the trunk.
   B. capillary haemangioma over the scalp.
   C. conjunctival telangiectases.
   D. café au lait spots.
   E. facial angiofibromas.

3. **An 8-month-old child is admitted after 48 hours of vomiting and diarrhoea. The baby's weight at a recent clinic visit was 8 kg. He is clinically estimated to be 10% dehydrated. Blood tests show isotonic dehydration:**
   A. there is a fluid deficit of 0.4 L.
   B. the blood gases will show a severe metabolic acidosis – pH < 7.2.
   C. A 20 ml/kg bolus of 0.9% saline is given immediately. The appropriate fluid for the next 24 hours would be 5% dextrose.
   D. *total* fluid requirement for the first 24 hours is approximately 2 L.
   E. skin turgor will be decreased.

4. **You have just given intravenous antibiotics to a child with cystic fibrosis. The child quickly becomes agitated, pale and loses consciousness. The blood pressure is unrecordable. Respiration is slow and gasping. There is no apparent wheeze, stridor or facial swelling. Appropriate emergency treatment would include:**
   A. oxygen.
   B. plasma 20 ml/kg by rapid infusion.
   C. intravenous calcium.
   D. intravenous adrenaline.
   E. intravenous 50% dextrose.

1. **BDE**

   In hydrocephalus a V-P shunt is extravascular and carries no risk of endocarditis. The risk of bacterial endocarditis is related to the presence of anatomical cardiac abnormality and associated turbulent blood flow. In atrial septal defects the very low pressure difference between the atria does not cause turbulent flow.

2. **AE**

   Cutaneous findings in tuberose sclerosis (TS) include a *shagreen* patch of rather coarse skin, depigmented macules and angiofibromas, a nodular eruption over the cheeks and bridge of the nose. Older children may develop subungual and periungual fibromas. TS is an autosomal dominant condition with a high new mutation rate. There is a strong association with epilepsy and a degree of mental retardation. Scalp capillary haemangiomas are associated with Sturge–Weber syndrome and conjunctival telangiectases with ataxia telangiectasia.

3. **DE**

   There is a fluid deficit of 0.8 L. Plasma or normal saline, 10–20 ml/kg, is given quickly to restore the circulating blood volume. The remainder of the fluid deficit, plus the normal (generous) daily fluid requirements (i.e. deficit of 800 ml + 150 ml/kg/day = 2 L), should be given over the next 24 hours. This will approximately correct the dehydration. Further fluid may need to be given if increased fluid loss continues. Decreased skin turgor and cool peripheries indicate 10% dehydration. Without hypotension or poor tissue perfusion, a metabolic acidosis is unlikely to develop. Dextrose 5% is not an appropriate resuscitation or maintenance fluid as hyponatraemia will develop.

4. **ABD**

   This is an acute anaphylactic reaction. ABCD of resuscitation. With no signs of airway obstruction and continuing respiratory effort, give 100% oxygen. Restore the circulation with volume – plasma – and most importantly, give specific treatment for this condition – *adrenaline*. Drugs may be given intravenously (IV). Without an available IV line, adrenaline should be given by deep IM injection. Cardiac massage, atropine and further adrenaline may be required if bradycardia or hypotension persist. Dextrose and calcium are unnecessary in this resuscitation.

5. **The following statements concerning forms of precocious puberty are true:**
   A. isolated breast development in an otherwise normal 2-year-old girl is likely to resolve spontaneously.
   B. enlargement of the penis without testicular enlargement suggests adrenal pathology.
   C. true precocious puberty is always accompanied by enlargement of the ovaries or testes.
   D. development of pubic hair and an increase in height velocity without other signs of secondary sexual characteristics indicate the onset of normal puberty.
   E. hypothyroidism is causally associated with precocious puberty.

6. **Intussusception:**
   A. occurs most commonly between 3 and 5 years of age.
   B. is most commonly ileocolic.
   C. is best treated by surgical reduction at laparotomy.
   D. is reliably diagnosed by ultrasound scan.
   E. is a recognised complication of Henoch Schönlein purpura.

7. **Features of the fetal alcohol syndrome include:**
   A. long, smooth philtrum.
   B. single palmar creases.
   C. ventricular septal defect.
   D. microcephaly.
   E. testicular enlargement.

8. **Delayed speech development is associated with:**
   A. bilateral hearing loss of 20 dB.
   B. autism.
   C. social isolation.
   D. no identifiable pathological cause in over 75%.
   E. fragile X syndrome.

5. **ABCE**

   Isolated transient thelarche (breast development) is relatively common in girls under 2 years and slightly raised FSH levels may be detected. If there are no other signs of pubertal development, investigation should be kept to a minimum but follow-up is essential. Enlargement of the testes and ovaries is the first sign of normal, pituitary (LH, FSH) driven onset of puberty. Enlargement of the penis alone suggests excessive androgen production. Hypo- *and* hyperthyroidism are both associated with precocious puberty.

6. **BDE**

   Intussusception occurs most commonly in the 3–9-month age range. Usually no predisposing cause is identified. The majority are ileocolic. Presentation is usually with severe colicky abdominal pain, and 60% may have blood in the stools, although this is a late sign. Air insufflation of the large bowel (an air enema) will usually reduce the intussusception. Unless there are signs of peritonism, surgery is rarely necessary. In Henoch Schönlein purpura mucosal bleeding may form the lead point for an intussusception. Ultrasound has no radiation hazard, is non-invasive, readily repeatable and is the imaging method of choice.

7. **ABCD**

   Alcohol is toxic to the developing brain with evidence of a dose–response effect. Intrauterine growth retardation with disproportionate microcephaly is typical of the severely affected neonate. Neonatal tremulousness or convulsions may occur. A number of dysmorphic features are common to the syndrome and include: single palmar crease, a long smooth philtrum with a thin upper lip; maxillary hypoplasia; short palpebral fissures and ptosis; facial hirsutism; and cardiac malformations. Testicular enlargement is seen in the fragile X syndrome, particularly after puberty.

8. **BCDE**

   Hearing loss of 40 dB is associated with difficulty hearing the normal spoken word. A hearing loss of only 20 dB would not constitute a significant hearing loss. Autism is commonly associated with absent or abnormal speech development. Fragile X syndrome is associated with mental retardation and often with speech delay. Emotionally neglected or socially isolated children may also show speech delay.

9. **In a child with recurrent episodes of loss of consciousness, the following would be more typical of a convulsion than a breath-holding spell:**
   A. tonic rigidity.
   B. age under 6 months.
   C. marked skin pallor.
   D. no history of precipitating event such as minor injury.
   E. sleepiness after the event, lasting for up to 1 hour.

10. **The following conditions are associated with a haemolytic anaemia:**
    A. sickle cell disease.
    B. iron deficiency.
    C. G6PD deficiency.
    D. beta-thalassaemia major.
    E. von Willebrand's disease.

11. **Complications of Group A Streptococcal infections include:**
    A. acute rheumatic fever.
    B. toxic shock syndrome.
    C. chorea.
    D. acute glomerulonephritis.
    E. Kawasaki disease.

12. **Bronchial lavage is carried out on a child who has a non-resolving pneumonia. *Mycobacterium tuberculosis* is isolated from the lavage sample:**
    A. the child is potentially infectious and should be excluded from school until the course of treatment is completed.
    B. Tuberculin skin testing of all family members and classmates is required.
    C. no treatment is required unless the Mantoux test is strongly positive.
    D. triple drug antituberculous therapy is given for 6 months.
    E. ethambutol should not be used for children under 5 years of age.

9. **BDE**

Breath-holding attacks occur in the toddler age group and follow a minor injury or temper tantrum. The child starts to cry, breath-holds and becomes purple in the face until either consciousness is lost or the episode resolves. Consciousness is quickly regained, there is no prolonged postictal period and no neurological deficit. A 'white' breath-holding spell is associated with profound pallor and loss of consciousness secondary to bradycardia or transient asystole. If significant hypoxia occurs, a short secondary convulsion may also occur. Tonic rigidity may occur in either a primary or secondary convulsion.

10. **ACD**

Congenital haemolysis may be caused by abnormalities of red cell shape (e.g. sphenocytosis), deficiency of red cell enzymes (e.g. G6PD deficiency) and is associated with the presence of unstable haemoglobins (HbS and Hb thal). Haemoglobinopathies result from genetically determined alteration in the globin polypeptide chain and may be diagnosed by haemoglobin electrophoresis.

11. **ACD**

Acute rheumatic fever, chorea and glomerulonephritis are all classical group A Streptococcal related conditions. Toxic shock syndrome is related to Staphylococcal infection, not only related to retained tampons but in children may be seen even with 'simple' infected eczema. No infectious agent has yet been isolated for Kawasaki disease.

12. **BE**

Open pulmonary TB (TB bacilli – AAFB – are seen on ZN stain of the sputum) is infectious. Children must be kept off school for 2 weeks after starting treatment, until the sputum becomes free of AAFB. A positive Mantoux test indicates that the child has either been exposed to TB in the past or has been immunised with BCG or has active infection. Contact tracing of all patients with open TB is vital for containment of the disease. The usual treatment for TB is with triple therapy (isoniazid, rifampicin and ethambutol) for 2 months, followed by 4 months of isoniazid and rifampicin together. Ethambutol should not be used in children under 5–6 years as it is important to be able to test colour vision during therapy.

13. **Neonatal necrotising enterocolitis:**
    A. occurs only in babies who have started milk feeding.
    B. can be prevented by the use of broad-spectrum antibiotics.
    C. is best treated by early excision of affected bowel.
    D. occurs only in babies who have had umbilical arterial catheters passed.
    E. requires treatment only if there are characteristic X-ray changes.

14. **A hypochloraemic hypokalaemic hyponatraemic metabolic alkalosis is found in:**
    A. pyloric stenosis.
    B. heat exhaustion in cystic fibrosis.
    C. Bartter's syndrome.
    D. severe (15%) dehydration.
    E. congential chloride-losing diarrhoea.

15. **At birth the majority of infants with an open mid-thoracic myelomeningocele with already have or will develop:**
    A. an associated hydrocephalus.
    B. a flaccid paralysis of both lower limbs.
    C. associated vertebral abnormalities.
    D. 'talipes' deformity of both feet.
    E. neonatal convulsions.

16. **A pulled elbow:**
    A. occurs in children aged between 5 and 10 years.
    B. shows as a hairline fracture of the radial head on X-ray.
    C. is painless.
    D. is typically held with the affected elbow flexed, forearm pronated and arm held tightly into the side.
    E. is treated with simple manipulation.

13. **None of these**

In necrotising enterocolitis (NEC) there is inflammation and invasion of the bowel wall by gas-producing organisms. Some infants who have never been fed enterally will develop NEC. Antibiotics do not prevent the condition. Feeding with expressed breast milk reduces the incidence of NEC. Operation is best delayed – it is difficult to determine bowel viability early in the disease. Treatment should be started if NEC is suspected (X-ray changes are not always present early in the disease) and includes stopping feeds, broad-spectrum antibiotics and parenteral nutrition. The aetiology is multifactorial and not solely related to the use of umbilical catheters.

14. **ABCE**

A child with 15% dehydration will be shocked with a (lactic) metabolic acidosis. In ABCE there is a problem with excessive chloride loss: pyloric stenosis – vomiting; cystic fibrosis – sweating; and Bartter's syndrome – renal loss. Low chloride levels restrict reabsorption of sodium in the proximal renal tubule. Sodium is presented to the distal renal tubule and is reabsorbed in exchange for hydrogen and potassium ions (under the influence of aldosterone).

15. **ACD**

Hydrocephalus will develop in 95% of babies with a thoracic myelomeningocele. Uncontrolled reflex activity can take place in an isolated segment of cord resulting in limb deformity. Reflex detrusor and sphincter muscle activity may or may not be coordinated. The bladder may be atonic, neurogenic or uncoordinated. The lower limbs may be flaccid or hypertonic. Hemivertebrae are common in high lesions and may cause kyphoscoliosis later in life. Neonatal convulsions are not a particular feature of spina bifida.

16. **DE**

A pulled elbow, subluxation of the radial head, is a common injury in the toddler age group and usually follows sudden traction on the hand with the elbow extended and forearm pronated. The child presents with an immobile arm held firmly to the side, with a flexed elbow and pronated forearm. Pain may be localised to the elbow or referred to the wrist or shoulder. X-rays do not show a fracture. Treatment is by gentle supination of the forearm with the arm in 90° flexion.

17. **All children admitted to hospital with moderate or severe asthma should have:**
    A. oral or intravenous steroid treatment.
    B. arterial blood gases.
    C. a chest X-ray.
    D. a sweat test.
    E. intravenous fluids at 150% of normal requirements.

18. **Features of Kawasaki disease include:**
    A. coronary arteritis.
    B. erosive arthritis.
    C. thrombocytosis.
    D. digital desquamation.
    E. purulent conjunctivitis.

19. **Inguinal hernia in infancy:**
    A. is commoner in boys than girls.
    B. affects right and left sides equally often.
    C. is bilateral in less than 10% of cases.
    D. affects relatively more ex-premature babies than full-term infants.
    E. should be electively repaired after the age of 6 months unless operation earlier is necessary because of incarceration or bowel obstruction.

20. **The following would be highly suggestive of non-accidental injury in an excessively drowsy 1-year-old child:**
    A. retinal haemorrhages.
    B. bulging fontanelle.
    C. haematuria.
    D. posterior rib fractures seen on chest X-ray.
    E. a depressed occipital skull fracture occurring after a fall off the parents' bed on to the floor.

**17.  A**
Any child admitted with asthma should be treated with anti-inflammatory doses of steroids. A capillary blood gas sample is better tolerated than a radial artery puncture and can be used for measurement of pH and $PCO_2$. Oxygen saturation is assessed by pulse oximetry. A chest X-ray is needed only if there is an abnormality on clinical examination – e.g. pneumothorax or failure to improve with treatment. A sweat test should be carried out only if there are atypical features. In asthma inappropriate ADH secretion may occur and pulmonary oedema may result from overgenerous intravenous fluid administration.

**18.  ACD**
Kawasaki disease is a vasculitic process characterised by a fever for more than 5 days, without demonstrable infective cause. Diagnostic features include: cervical lymphadenopathy, a non-purulent conjunctivitis, an erythematous rash, redness and swelling of the hands and feet followed by peeling of the digits, inflammation of the lips and buccal mucosa, and a strawberry tongue. Coronary arteritis and coronary artery aneurysms may develop in up to 20% of untreated cases. Thrombocytosis and a high ESR are common findings.

**19.  AD**
Inguinal hernias are much commoner in boys than girls (90% vs 10%). Hernias occur most frequently on the right (70%) and are bilateral in approximately 10–15% of cases. Hernias occur relatively more frequently in ex-preterm infants, but ex-prems comprise only 25% of infants requiring surgery. Hernias should be repaired as soon as is clinically convenient to minimise the risk of bowel strangulation.

**20.  ADE**
A bulging fontanelle and haematuria are non-specific signs. Posterior rib fractures usually result from chest compression by adult hands encircling the chest. Chest compression producing acutely raised central venous pressure often also causes retinal haemorrhages. A depressed occipital fracture is itself highly suggestive of abuse. Accidental skull fractures tend to be single, parietal, crack fractures. A skull fracture rarely (if ever) results from a fall from a low bed. Falls documented from hospital cots on to hard floors very rarely result in skull fractures.

# 16

## Ophthalmology and otolaryngology

1. **When assessing vision in a preschool child:**
   A. a 2-year-old can cooperate with the use of a Snellen chart.
   B. a normal pupillary light reflex excludes a significant visual defect.
   C. the human face is the best object to encourage a baby to fix and follow.
   D. parental concern about an infant's vision should always be treated seriously.
   E. observing visual fixation on moving balls of various sizes can be employed from 6 months of age.

2. **When assessing a child with a suspected squint:**
   A. the squint may be apparent only when looking in one direction.
   B. a convergent squint describes a malaligned eye which is turned out.
   C. a broad nasal bridge can create the illusion of a convergent squint.
   D. during the cover test, movement of the eye to take up fixation (after the eye is uncovered) excludes the presence of a squint.
   E. an intermittent squint in a toddler can be safely ignored.

3. **Regarding squints:**
   A. a fixed squint in a 1-month-old baby does not require investigation.
   B. all children with a squint should have their visual acuity tested.
   C. in 90% of cases, a specific cause can be identified.
   D. patching of the non-squinting eye is more likely to be effective at school age than in infancy.
   E. failure to correct the squint in early life causes permanent visual impairment in the affected eye.

4. **The following conditions cause cataracts:**
   A. Down syndrome.
   B. diabetes insipidus.
   C. Duchenne muscular dystrophy.
   D. congenital rubella.
   E. retinoblastoma.

1. **CDE**

   The Snellen chart employs letters of graded size to determine visual acuity and is suitable for children of 7 years or older. Testing vision in young infants is limited to observation of visual fixation on a face or object, or ability to turn towards a light source. The Stycar graded balls test involves observation of the subject's ability to fix and follow moving balls of various sizes at various distances. Normal pupil response is a brainstem reflex and gives no other information about vision. Parents' concerns should always be taken seriously.

2. **AC**

   A subtle squint may be apparent only when the child looks in a particular direction or is observed closely. A broad nasal bridge or epicanthic folds can create the illusion of a squint. A latent squint may be revealed by the cover test. A convergent squint turns the affected eye inward towards the nose. Intermittent squints are common in the first few months of life but should always be assessed fully after 6 months of age.

3. **BE**

   A fixed squint at any age and intermittent squints persisting beyond 6 months of age should be referred to an ophthalmologist. Hypermetropia, myopia and astigmatism can cause a squint but, in most cases, no specific cause is found. Untreated irreversible failure of visual function on the affected side (amblyopia) can develop. Treatment involves correction of any treatable lesion, then covering the 'good' eye which stimulates the use of the amblyopic eye; this is more effective in infancy.

4. **AD**

   Cataracts may be idiopathic or familial. Specific causes of cataract include congenital infections, Down syndrome, myotonic dystrophy, diabetes mellitus and some inborn errors of metabolism. An abnormality of the red reflex (the light reflected from the ophthalmoscope off the retina) may indicate a cataract is present; retinoblastoma is another cause of loss of the red reflex. Checking for the red reflex is part of the routine neonatal examination.

5. **Regarding conjunctivitis in childhood:**
    A. *Neisseria gonorrhoeae* is effectively treated with topical antibiotics.
    B. Chlamydia conjunctivitis is associated with respiratory infection in infancy.
    C. in school-age children, the commonest aetiology is bacterial infection.
    D. Herpes simplex infection can present with viral conjunctivitis.
    E. topical steroids are first-line treatment for allergic conjunctivitis.

6. **Blindness:**
    A. is genetically determined in less than 5% of childhood cases in the UK.
    B. due to retinopathy of prematurity, can be completely prevented if oxygen therapy is properly regulated.
    C. must be suspected in a 4-month-old infant with roving eye movements.
    D. in children is amenable to medical intervention in over 50% of cases.
    E. after measles is commoner in developing countries because of vitamin C deficiency.

7. **Retinoblastoma:**
    A. occurs in 1:2000 live births.
    B. goes into spontaneous remission in 30% of cases.
    C. has an autosomal dominant inheritance in 40% of cases.
    D. has an excellent prognosis if there is early diagnosis and adequate treatment.
    E. requires surgical removal of the eye in the majority of sporadic cases.

8. **Regarding normal development of vision:**
    A. response to light is present from the 7th month of pregnancy.
    B. an infant can discriminate a number of parental facial expressions within 48 hours of birth.
    C. binocular vision is well established at 4 weeks of age.
    D. mild myopia (near sightedness) is a normal finding in infancy and early childhood.
    E. visual acuity is equal to normal adult values by 1 year of age.

5.  **BD**

    Conjunctivitis is a common problem in childhood. Neonatal conjunctivitis may be acquired from the birth canal. *Neisseria gonorrhoeae* infection threatens sight and requires treatment with intravenous antibiotic. Perinatally acquired Chlamydia can cause conjunctivitis and pneumonia. In older children the commonest aetiology is viral infection. Allergic conjunctivitis in atopic individuals is also common and can be treated with topical antihistamine or sodium cromoglycate. Topical steroids are reserved for severe cases.

6.  **C**

    Normal children stop showing uncoordinated eye movements by 6 weeks of age. Roving eye movements or pendular nystagmus must raise the suspicion of blindness. In the UK around 50% of blindness in childhood is genetically determined. Some cataracts can be treated, but there is no treatment for most causes of blindness. The aetiology of retinopathy of prematurity is multifactorial, so some preterm infants will develop visual impairment despite careful regulation of oxygen therapy. Vitamin A deficiency predisposes to failure of corneal repair after measles; dietary supplements may prevent this complication.

7.  **CDE**

    Retinoblastoma is a rare tumour; the incidence is around 1:20 000 live births. About 40% of cases are familial with an autosomal dominant inheritance. Familial cases should be detected early by regular ophthalmic examination. Sporadic cases tend to present with more advanced disease and removal of the eye is usually necessary. With early diagnosis and treatment, mortality is below 5%, but untreated retinoblastoma is invariably fatal.

8.  **AB**

    The fetus responds to light by 7 months' gestation. Newborns can focus on a human face and are able to respond to changing facial expressions. Binocular vision becomes established between 3 and 6 months of age. 'Adult' visual acuity is present from around 4 years of age. Normal infants are slightly hypermetropic (long sighted) and this tendency persists until adolescence, when there is usually no refractive error. In adult life there is a tendency to myopia (near sightedness).

9. **Regarding congenital malformations of the eye:**
   A. microphthalmia is likely to be associated with visual impairment in the affected eye.
   B. a coloboma is an opacification of the lens.
   C. colobomas are associated with multiple congenital malformations.
   D. identification of optic nerve hypoplasia should lead to investigation for endocrine deficiencies.
   E. aniridia is associated with the development of Wilms tumour (nephroblastoma).

10. **Bilateral choanal atresia:**
    A. presents in the neonatal period.
    B. particularly causes difficulties for newborn infants because they are obligate nose breathers.
    C. requires an artificial airway to be passed.
    D. can be confirmed using nasal endoscopy.
    E. requires surgical repair.

11. **Acute sinusitis:**
    A. is common in the 1st year of life.
    B. is diagnosed with plain radiographs.
    C. causes tenderness over the affected sinuses.
    D. is caused by *Streptococcus pneumoniae*.
    E. can be complicated by orbital cellulitis.

12. **Cleft palate:**
    A. rarely causes difficulty with feeding in infancy.
    B. occurs in 1:10 000 births.
    C. is associated with a chromosomal abnormality in the majority of cases.
    D. should be repaired between 3 and 4 years of age.
    E. is associated with recurrent serous otitis media.

9.  **ACDE**

    There is a range of degree of microphthalmia (impaired growth of the ocular structures); some visual impairment is usual. A coloboma occurs when there is a failure of closure of the optic cup in embryogenesis. This results in a segmental defect in ocular structures at one or more levels; these may include defects in the eyelid, iris, retina or optic nerve. Colobomas are commonly associated with syndromes of congenital malformations. Optic nerve hypoplasia is a component of septo-optic dysplasia, an abnormality which involves visual impairment and hypopituitarism.

10. **ABCDE**

    Choanal atresia is a developmental anomaly in which the nasal passages are obstructed. Since infants are obligate nasal breathers, bilateral atresia presents soon after birth with respiratory distress and cyanosis. A temporary airway is passed until surgical repair can be performed.

11. **CDE**

    Maxillary and ethmoid sinuses are present at birth, the sphenoids develop around 3 years and the frontal sinuses about 6 years. Sinus disease is uncommon in early childhood. Diagnosis can be difficult. Tenderness over the affected site is useful. Plain radiographs sometimes demonstrate a fluid level, but can be difficult to interpret. CT scans can be helpful. Respiratory pathogens are usually responsible. Acute sinusitis can be complicated by orbital cellulitis, cavernous sinus thrombosis and intracranial sepsis.

12. **E**

    Cleft lip and palate are caused by a combination of genetic factors and unknown environmental influences. A family history is common but, in most cases, there is no other abnormality present. The defect is common; cleft lip or palate occurs in 1:600 births. Various elements of the mid-facial skeleton are affected, including the Eustachian tubes which are prone to obstruction. Repair is usually carried out before 1 year, often in the first 6 months.

13. **The following are valid indications of tonsillectomy:**
    A. four episodes of sore throat in 1 year.
    B. frequent episodes of purulent tonsillitis leading to time lost from school.
    C. gross tonsillar hypertrophy due to infectious mononucleosis.
    D. an episode of quinsy.
    E. obstructive sleep apnoea with tonsillar hypertrophy.

14. **In the evaluation of possible obstructive sleep apnoea:**
    A. the presence of Down syndrome increases the likelihood of a positive diagnosis.
    B. overnight measurement of oxygen saturation is valuable.
    C. a history of loud snoring is irrelevant.
    D. a history of restlessness during sleep excludes the diagnosis.
    E. a history of early morning vomiting is consistent with this diagnosis.

15. **Laryngomalacia:**
    A. is due to abnormally compliant laryngeal cartilage.
    B. is characterised by stridor which develops around 2 years of age.
    C. causes lifelong symptoms in the majority of cases.
    D. requires endoscopic confirmation, even in mild cases.
    E. requires tracheostomy in around 20% of cases.

16. **With regard to conditions causing chronic stridor:**
    A. in unilateral vocal cord palsy, progressive improvement of the stridor with age is likely.
    B. surgical clearance of laryngeal papillomas is rarely possible.
    C. subglottic stenosis is associated with prolonged endotracheal intubation in infancy.
    D. a subglottic haemangioma should always be surgically excised.
    E. most preschool children can cooperate with a diagnostic direct laryngoscopy.

13. **BDE**

Pharyngitis is a common infection in childhood. Tonsillitis is usually due to bacterial infection in the tonsillar crypts. Acute tonsillar enlargement is seen in infectious mononucleosis, but this is an acute, self-limiting disorder. Children with adeno-tonsillar hypertrophy may develop obstructive sleep apnoea and surgery is needed to relieve the obstruction. Quinsy is a peri-tonsillar abscess and tonsillectomy is usually performed after the acute infection has resolved.

14. **AB**

During normal sleep, there is reduced pharyngeal muscle tone which makes the upper airway prone to collapse during inspiration. If the airway is further narrowed by an anatomical abnormality (e.g. Down syndrome) or by adeno-tonsillar hypertrophy, there may be intermittent, complete upper airway obstruction. This manifests as loud snoring, restless sleep and resultant daytime drowsiness. The diagnosis is made from the history and by identifying airway obstruction during a sleep study. Significant hypoxia during sleep indicates the need for urgent treatment.

15. **A**

Laryngomalacia is due to collapse of compliant laryngeal cartilage and low-placed epiglottis. The condition presents within weeks of birth with intermittent stridor associated with crying and exertion. It is a self-limiting condition and intervention is virtually never required. Stridor usually resolves before 18 months of age. In most cases, a clinical diagnosis can be made. If there is stridor during quiet breathing or evidence of respiratory compromise, direct laryngoscopy is indicated.

16. **ABC**

Diagnosis of the cause of chronic upper airway obstruction requires laryngoscopy, usually under general anaesthetic in children. Laryngeal papillomatosis is a condition where virus-induced warts develop on the vocal cords. Surgical clearance is rarely possible, but spontaneous recovery occurs in some cases. Subglottic stenosis may be congenital or caused by chronic intubation, particularly in infancy. Subglottic haemangiomas, like cavernous haemangiomas, enlarge initially and regress in later childhood. Surgical intervention is best avoided. If there is airway compromise, tracheostomy may be required.

**17. The following are causes of conductive hearing loss in a child:**
   A. perinatal asphyxia.
   B. congenital cytomegalovirus infection.
   C. severe unconjugated hyperbilirubinaemia in the neonatal period.
   D. exposure to toxic levels of aminoglycoside antibiotic.
   E. serous otitis media.

**18. The following are indications for a formal hearing assessment:**
   A. parental concern that the child cannot hear normally.
   B. premature birth at 35 weeks' gestation.
   C. a family history of hearing impairment.
   D. failure to speak more than six words by 14 months of age.
   E. an episode of bacterial meningitis.

**19. Acute suppurative otitis media:**
   A. is diagnosed by pneumatic otoscopy.
   B. commonly presents with fever and irritability in preschool children.
   C. causes pain which worsens if the tympanic membrane perforates.
   D. if complicated by facial palsy, indicates that a mastoiditis is present.
   E. is most commonly caused by *Pseudomonas aeruginosa*.

**20. A child with serous otitis media:**
   A. is likely to present with insidious onset hearing loss.
   B. will benefit from antibiotic ear-drops.
   C. will have impaired movement of the tympanic membrane.
   D. may have air–fluid levels or air bubbles which may be seen behind the tympanic membrane on otoscopy.
   E. a middle ear drainage tube (grommet) should be inserted routinely as early as possible.

17. **E**

All of these conditions cause sensorineural deafness except serous otitis media.

18. **ACE**

A number of risk factors for hearing impairment should lead to careful hearing assessment. These factors include parental concerns about hearing, familial deafness and exposure to ototoxic factors such as aminoglycosides, high levels of bilirubin and certain infections (e.g. Cytomegalovirus). Premature infants born before 33 weeks' gestation are at increased risk of hearing impairment. Speech delay is an important indication for audiological assessment, but concern about failure to speak six words would not be significant before the age of 2 years.

19. **BD**

Older children can report earache but in young children otitis media will present with non-specific features of a febrile illness. Simple otoscopy establishes the diagnosis, revealing a bulging, inflamed tympanic membrane or pus in the auditory canal if the membrane has ruptured. Serous otitis media is diagnosed by pneumatic otoscopy. The pain of otitis media is due to pressure on the tympanic membrane and improves if the membrane ruptures. Extension of the infection to the adjacent mastoid bone is a dangerous complication, manifested by tenderness, facial palsy, labyrinthitis or signs of intracranial abscess. Otitis media is usually caused by pathogens such as Streptococci, Staphylococci or *Haemophilus influenzae*.

20. **ACD**

In serous otitis media (glue ear) there is a chronic middle ear effusion without infection. The aetiology is incompletely understood, but the anatomy of the middle ear in children, and infection and allergy, may all be contributory. In some cases there is discomfort, but many cases present with hearing impairment observed by parents, teachers or detected at routine screening. The effusion impairs movement of the tympanic membrane, observed during pneumatic otoscopy. The value of grommet insertion is being re-evaluated. Some cases are self-limiting and treatment is not needed.

# 17

# Growth and Endocrinology

1. **Growth hormone deficiency:**
   A. presents with short stature and poor weight gain.
   B. is treated with a weekly injection of growth hormone.
   C. is diagnosed by MRI scan of pituitary.
   D. is caused by lack of production of growth hormone by the posterior pituitary.
   E. results in an advanced bone age for chronological age.

2. **Indications of panhypopituitarism in a neonate are:**
   A. hyperglycaemia.
   B. enlarged genitalia.
   C. prolonged jaundice.
   D. hypothermia.
   E. severe intra-uterine growth retardation.

3. **Hypoglycaemia in the normal neonate:**
   A. stimulates liver glycogenolysis and gluconeogenesis.
   B. causes glucagon levels to fall.
   C. occurs because of the cessation of transplacental glucose delivery.
   D. is not a concern unless the blood glucose level is less than 1.0 mmol/L.
   E. suppresses any insulin production.

4. **Female pseudohermaphrodites:**
   A. have XY karyotype.
   B. have virilisation of the external genitalia.
   C. result from excess androgen exposure.
   D. should be screened for congenital adrenal hyperplasia.
   E. have normal ovaries and Mullerian structures.

1. **None of these – all false**
   Growth hormone is produced by the anterior pituitary gland in pulses during the night. Deficiency classically presents with short stature and obesity in the 2nd or 3rd year of life. The diagnosis is confirmed by stimulating the pituitary gland to produce growth hormone during a provocation test. Imaging of the pituitary is important, either to exclude a tumour or to determine congenital abnormalities of the gland, but it is not diagnostic. The treatment is with daily growth hormone injections, usually given in the evening. The bone age is delayed.

2. **CD**
   The pituitary gland produces growth hormone, ACTH, LH, FSH, TSH, ADH and oxytocin. Absence of the gland usually causes problems with anterior pituitary hormone production. The neonate may be hypoglycaemic and cold as growth hormone and cortisol are important counter-regulatory hormones that stimulate glucose production. Prolonged jaundice may indicate central hypothyroidism. The genitalia are classically small as the LH/FSH axis is active in utero. These babies are not usually small as growth in utero is more dependent upon placental function.

3. **AE**
   Hypoglycaemia in the neonate is thought to have detrimental effects on neurological function. Hypoglycaemia is defined as a blood glucose level less than 2.6 mmol/L. In utero the glucose supply is across the placenta. Postnatally the infant has to switch on mechanisms to convert body stores laid down in the third trimester into energy until milk intake is established. Glucagon levels rise and stimulate gluconeogenesis and glycogenolysis. Insulin production is suppressed.

4. **BCDE**
   A female infant (XX karyotype), if exposed to excess androgens in utero, will have virilisation of the external genitalia – a female pseudohermaphrodite. The internal structures are normal. The commonest cause is due to congenital adrenal hyperplasia, typically 21-hydroxylase deficiency. There may be significant virilisation and surgery may be required for clitoral reduction and vaginal reconstruction.

5.  **A baby with XY karyotype has ambiguous genitalia. The causes to consider are:**
    A.  impaired peripheral androgen metabolism.
    B.  Sertoli cell hypoplasia.
    C.  abnormality in production of Mullerian inhibitory hormone.
    D.  congenital adrenal hyperplasia.
    E.  Klinefelter syndrome.

6.  **The management of a baby with ambiguous genitalia includes:**
    A.  gender assignment within the 1st week of birth.
    B.  urgent karyotype.
    C.  serum electrolytes.
    D.  17-hydroxy-progesterone level.
    E.  clinical examination for testes.

7.  **Hypothalamic diabetes insipidus:**
    A.  presents with polyuria only if the sensation of thirst is preserved.
    B.  is the presenting feature of Langerhans cell histiocytosis in 20–30% of cases.
    C.  results from renal unresponsiveness to antidiuretic hormone.
    D.  may present with hypernatraemic dehydration.
    E.  is unlikely if the child has nocturia.

8.  **Inappropriate antidiuretic hormone secretion:**
    A.  results in low urinary sodium concentration.
    B.  causes dilutional hyponatraemia.
    C.  stimulates secretion of aldosterone.
    D.  is seen in 50% of severely asphyxiated babies.
    E.  occurs in 20% of children with meningitis.

5.  **ACD**

    Impaired peripheral androgen metabolism is the commonest cause of ambiguous genitalia and includes complete and incomplete androgen insensitivity syndromes. Complete testicular feminisation may only present at puberty with primary amenorrhoea. Rare causes include Leydig cell hypoplasia and abnormality in Mullerian inhibitory hormone, so that Fallopian tubes and uterus are present usually in a fairly virilised male. The rarer types of congenital adrenal hyperplasia may cause a defect in androgen production.

6.  **BCDE**

    The sex assigned to a child is not dependent on the karyotype, but on the diagnosis and the possibility of future sexual function. Gender assignment and birth registration should be deferred for as long as necessary. The child with ambiguous genitalia should have the 17-hydroxy progesterone level and serum electrolytes checked because of the risk of a salt-losing crisis. An urgent karyotype can take 48 hours. The presence of palpable gonads (probably testes) will aid the clinical diagnosis of the genetic sex.

7.  **ABD**

    Hypothalamic DI is due to failure of production of antidiuretic hormone. The renal tubules do not therefore have the stimulus to produce concentrated urine. Large volumes of dilute urine are passed and dehydration results unless there is compensatory high intake of fluid. In some cases, the thirst sensation is lost and hypernatraemic dehydration results. Because of the large volumes of urine, nocturia is always present. It is the presenting feature of LCH in 20–30% of cases and may occur many years before other symptoms.

8.  **BDE**

    The syndrome of inappropriate antidiuretic hormone secretion (SIADH) can be triggered by a wide variety of pathologies. The principal stimulus to ADH release is a rise in plasma osmolarity which results in concentrated urine and dilute plasma. ADH acts to increase water reabsorption by the distal renal tubules and collecting ducts. High ADH levels inhibit the production of aldosterone. SIADH occurs in many conditions, including severe birth asphyxia and meningitis.

9. **A 9-year-old girl is found to have a craniopharyngioma:**
   A. presentation with precocious puberty may occur.
   B. a homonymous hemianopia may be found on testing visual fields.
   C. urgent surgical resection is required.
   D. admission for hypothalamic-pituitary function tests should be arranged.
   E. investigation for metastatic spread is required.

10. **Congenital hypothyroidism:**
    A. occurs in 1 in 10 000 births.
    B. has an increased incidence in infants with Down syndrome.
    C. is most commonly caused by inborn errors of thyroid hormone biosynthesis.
    D. is always detectable by screening at days 5–7 on dried blood spot.
    E. is not associated with developmental delay if treatment is initiated within the first 12 weeks of life.

11. **A 2-week-old baby is thought to have hypothyroidism because of the following clinical features:**
    A. microglossia.
    B. prolonged jaundice.
    C. diarrhoea.
    D. maternal Graves' disease.
    E. wide posterior fontanelle.

12. **Serum calcium levels are:**
    A. increased by parathyroid hormone mobilising calcium from bone.
    B. decreased by vitamin D action on distal renal tubule absorption.
    C. high in nutritional rickets.
    D. increased by vitamin D mediated absorption from intestinal villi.
    E. low in calcitonin hypersecretion.

**9. D**

A craniopharyngioma is the commonest tumour affecting the hypothalamic-pituitary region in children. The tumours are benign but progressive local enlargement results in significant pathology. Compression of the optic chiasm results in visual disturbance. Pituitary destruction resulting in hormone deficiencies may present with delayed growth and puberty in the adolescent. Hormone and neurological function should be assessed before treatment. Surgery is only urgent if there are significant visual or neurological disturbances. Surgery will exacerbate any endocrine deficit and total excision is usually impossible.

**10. B**

The incidence is 1 in 4000. In the UK it is screened for on the Guthrie card at 5–7 days. All cases are not detected because 1 in 100 cases will be due to hypothalamic-pituitary problems and therefore the TSH will not be elevated. The screen relies on an elevated TSH. There is an increased incidence in Down syndrome and other trisomies. The majority of cases are due to thyroid dysgenesis. Treatment must be started within the first few weeks in order to prevent neurological damage.

**11. BE**

Babies with congenital hypothyroidism are often placid, sleepy babies, who feed poorly, have umbilical herniae, large tongues, wide posterior fontanelle, prolonged jaundice, constipation, hypothermia, peripheral cyanosis and oedema. Maternal Graves' disease may cause transient hyperthyroidism in a baby if maternal thyroid-stimulating antibodies cross the placenta.

**12. AD**

Serum calcium levels are controlled by vitamin D, parathyroid hormone (PTH) and calcitonin. Vitamin D increases serum calcium by stimulating intestinal absorption and mobilisation from bone and reducing renal excretion. PTH prevents hypocalcaemia by stimulating calcium mobilisation from bone and increasing calcium reabsorption from renal tubules, and stimulates renal vitamin D synthesis. Nutritional rickets results in low serum calcium, so stimulating bone mobilisation. Although calcitonin does regulate calcium levels, hypersecretion does not cause hypocalcaemia.

13. **In primary hyperparathyroidism:**
    A. a parathyroid adenoma is the likely cause.
    B. the presenting feature can be a pathological fracture.
    C. ureteric colic is due to calcium stones.
    D. hypercalcaemia with low levels of parathormone is diagnostic.
    E. polyuria and polydipsia are compensatory mechanisms.

14. **The presenting features of pseudohypoparathyroidism are:**
    A. due to a defect in receptor at the target organ.
    B. with high serum levels of parathormone.
    C. hypercalcaemia.
    D. mental retardation.
    E. absent thumbs.

15. **Rickets may be due to:**
    A. lack of sunshine.
    B. coeliac disease.
    C. excessive urinary phosphate excretion.
    D. chronic renal failure.
    E. lack of vitamin A.

16. **In congenital adrenal hyperplasia due to 21-hydroxylase deficiency:**
    A. presentation is with low ACTH.
    B. the inheritance is autosomal dominant.
    C. there is incomplete virilisation of male genitalia.
    D. antenatal diagnosis is possible for the first born.
    E. there is a defect in mineralocorticoid biosynthesis in 50–75% of cases.

13. **ABCE**

Primary hyperparathyroidism is rare at 2–5 per 100 000. The commonest cause is a parathyroid adenoma. High PTH levels raise serum calcium levels causing non-specific symptoms such as lethargy, anorexia and constipation. The calcium is mobilised from bone which may become osteopenic and susceptible to fracture. Renal calculi develop – polyuria and polydipsia are compensatory mechanisms in an attempt to lower the serum calcium level.

14. **ABD**

Pseudohypoparathyroidism results from end-organ resistance to parathyroid hormone (PTH). Therefore there are high levels of PTH but hypocalcaemia as the target organs are not stimulated to increase the serum level. These people have characteristic phenotypic features – short stature, short 4th and 5th metacarpals and obesity with a round face and short neck. They also have variable mental retardation.

15. **ABCD**

Failure of vitamin D absorption from the proximal small intestine may occur in coeliac disease causing rickets. Vitamin D can be synthesised in the skin. A diet low in vitamin D and minimal exposure to sunlight are risk factors for the development of rickets. Vitamin D resistant rickets, an X-linked dominant characteristic, is due to excessive urinary phosphate excretion. Chronic renal failure may cause rickets due to failure of vitamin D hydroxylation. Vitamin A deficiency does not cause rickets.

16. **E**

The adrenal cortex synthesises mineralocorticoids, glucocorticoids and androgens. Congenital adrenal hyperplasia results in a build up of metabolites, proximal to the enzyme block, which are diverted down other pathways resulting in an excess of some hormones. The commonest enzyme deficiency is 21-hydroxylase. It presents with high ACTH levels due to loss of negative cortisol feedback. Inheritance is autosomal recessive. Antenatal diagnosis is possible for subsequent pregnancies. 21-hydroxylase enzyme deficiency results in all cases in glucocorticoid deficiency, but with mineralocorticoid deficiency in 50–75% of cases.

17. **Clinical features that suggest a diagnosis of congenital adrenal hyperplasia in a female infant are:**
    A. collapse with hypernatraemic dehydration.
    B. labio-scrotal fold fusion.
    C. genital pigmentation.
    D. delayed bone age.
    E. hypertension.

18. **Excess of steroids, either iatrogenic or endogenous causes:**
    A. protein anabolism.
    B. hypotension.
    C. centripetal obesity.
    D. hirsutism.
    E. growth failure.

19. **The causes of Cushing syndrome are:**
    A. congenital adrenal hypoplasia.
    B. an adrenal carcinoma.
    C. growth hormone insufficiency.
    D. pituitary ACTH hypersecretion.
    E. oral administration of glucocorticoid.

20. **Addison's disease:**
    A. occurs in 1 in 10 000 children.
    B. is associated with mucocutaneous candidiasis.
    C. presents with hyperglycaemia.
    D. results in hypokalaemia.
    E. causes excess sweating.

## 17.  BCE

Excess of androgens results in virilisation of a female infant. There may be labio-scrotal fold fusion. A lack of mineralo-corticoid may cause collapse with hyponatraemic dehydration. Excess pigmentation results from the high ACTH level that also stimulates the melanocyte-stimulating hormone. Bone age is classically advanced because of the excess androgens. If the enzyme block leads to excess mineralocorticoid production, then the baby would be hypertensive.

## 18.  CDE

Steroid excess results in protein catabolism, increased carbo-hydrate metabolism, fat accumulation and potassium loss. In children the most consistent features are progressive truncal obesity, growth failure and hirsutism. Other features are hypertension, striae and muscle weakness.

## 19.  BDE

Any cause of excess glucocorticoid will result in Cushing's syndrome. An adrenal carcinoma may produce excess amounts. Pituitary hypersecretion of ACTH will cause excess adrenal steroid production. Oral administration will result in the same features. Congenital adrenal hypoplasia results in deficiency of glucocorticoid. Growth hormone insufficiency does not cause Cushing's syndrome.

## 20.  AB

Primary adrenal insufficiency occurs in 1 in 10 000 children. The commonest cause is autoimmune disease, and there is an association with other autoimmune diseases, including muco-cutaneous candidiasis. The symptoms result from cortisol and aldosterone deficiency. Severe hypoglycaemia may occur in times of stress; hyponatraemia and hyperkalaemia result from aldosterone deficiency. This may be exacerbated by ADH production due to decreased plasma volume. ACTH causes melanocyte stimulation – buccal mucosa and palmar creases are the common sites of pigmentation.

21. **Insulin:**
    A. stimulates gluconeogenesis.
    B. inhibits glucose uptake by fat and muscle cells.
    C. stimulates amino acid incorporation into muscle protein.
    D. production is increased by glucose and amino acids.
    E. is produced at twice the rate of C-peptide.

22. **Glucagon:**
    A. is produced in the islet beta cells of the pancreas.
    B. production is increased by starvation.
    C. stimulates glycogenolysis.
    D. increases free fatty acid level in blood.
    E. levels are increased by insulin.

23. **The classical presenting features of diabetes mellitus are:**
    A. weight gain.
    B. polydipsia.
    C. enuresis.
    D. constipation.
    E. recurrent infections.

24. **A child presents in a collapsed state. The features that indicate diabetic ketoacidosis include:**
    A. hypoventilation.
    B. severe abdominal pain with guarding.
    C. metabolic acidosis.
    D. anuria.
    E. hypokalaemia.

21. **CD**

Insulin stimulates glucose and amino acid uptake into fat and muscle cells and conversion to glycogen and triglycerides. It inhibits lipolysis, glycogenolysis, gluconeogenesis and muscle breakdown. The production of insulin is increased by circulating glucose and amino acids. It is produced as pro-insulin which is cleaved to form insulin and C-peptide. The production of both is therefore the same.

22. **BCD**

Glucagon is produced in the alpha cells. The production of glucagon is increased in times of starvation and hypoglycaemia. It stimulates glycogenolysis, gluconeogenesis and fat cell lipolysis, so increasing free fatty acids and ketones. Glucagon levels are suppressed by insulin.

23. **BC**

A newly presenting diabetic will usually have lost weight. They are unable to utilise glucose. They rely on body stores for energy. The high serum glucose causes an osmotic diuresis. The children therefore have polydipsia and polyuria, with large amounts of glucose in the urine. They do not present with recurrent infections, although it is usually necessary to exclude a urinary tract infection.

24. **BC**

Diabetic ketoacidosis occurs in the newly presenting diabetic or in a poorly controlled diabetic. Ketosis occurs as fat stores are broken down to provide energy while glucose cannot be utilised. Dehydration occurs as the hyperglycaemia causes an osmotic diuresis. Ketosis causes vomiting. Oral fluids are not tolerated. There may be severe abdominal pain with guarding. This resolves as the metabolic derangement is corrected. Deep and sighing respirations occur in an attempt to counter the metabolic acidosis. Hypokalaemia is uncommon due to shift of potassium from the intracellular to extracellular space. Total body potassium is low.

25. **The incidence of type 1 diabetes mellitus:**
    A. has seasonal variation.
    B. is the same for identical and non-identical twins.
    C. is consistent world-wide at approximately 10 per 100 000.
    D. is increased in people who express DR3 or DR4, or both of these antigens.
    E. is decreased in populations who immunise against influenza.

26. **The ideal monitoring of the established diabetic:**
    A. daily urine test for ketones.
    B. blood glucose level 30 min to 1 hour after each meal and before bed.
    C. assessment of HbAlc levels 6-monthly.
    D. fundoscopy yearly.
    E. yearly screening for coeliac disease.

27. **Regarding insulin:**
    A. the dose should be increased prior to exercise.
    B. the injection should be omitted if the child is vomiting.
    C. requirements decrease during puberty.
    D. endogenous production can be monitored with C-peptide levels.
    E. absorption varies with site injected (excluding areas of lipohypertrophy).

28. **Blood should be taken at the time of hypoglycaemia to aid diagnosis. The request to the lab should include:**
    A. glucose level.
    B. ketones.
    C. growth hormone.
    D. reducing substances.
    E. lactate.

25.  **AD**

There is a genetic predisposition to diabetes mellitus. 98% of all type I insulin-dependent diabetics express DR3 or DR4, or both of these antigens. However, less than 1% of healthy subjects with these markers will develop diabetes. The risk is increased for a second twin. The incidence varies worldwide and increases with increasing distance from the equator. There is a seasonal variation. It is suggested that a virus may trigger autoimmune destruction in susceptible individuals.

26.  **DE**

The insulin requirements should be monitored with blood glucose measurements prior to administration. Daily urine ketone measurement is unnecessary and will only be positive at times of poor control or illness. The HbAlc level gives an idea of blood glucose control over the previous 6–8 weeks. Fundoscopy should be done yearly, particularly after puberty. Diabetes is associated with an increased incidence of coeliac disease.

27.  **DE**

Insulin doses should not be omitted. If a child is unable to take oral food or fluids, they may require admission. Insulin doses may need to be reduced prior to exercise or extra snacks taken as exercise will mobilise stores of insulin from fat. During puberty, insulin requirements increase. Diabetes may be harder to control due to psychological problems and also to the development of relative growth hormone resistance. In newly diagnosed diabetics some insulin production may be retained. This can be monitored by measuring C-peptide levels. Insulin absorption varies with the injection site – quicker from arms than abdomen, and slower from thighs.

28.  **ABCE**

It is very important to take blood samples at the time of hypoglycaemia when there should be appropriate suppression of insulin and elevation of the counter-regulatory hormones such as growth hormone. There should be evidence of a normal metabolic response with the breakdown of fats to form free fatty acids and ketones, of proteins to form amino acids and utilisation of lactate for energy. The urine should be checked for reducing substances.

**29. Causes of ketotic hypoglycaemia include:**
A. growth hormone deficiency.
B. insulinoma.
C. Addison's disease.
D. congenital adrenal hyperplasia.
E. defect in beta oxidation of fatty acids.

**30. The causes of non-ketotic hypoglycaemia include:**
A. galactosaemia.
B. Reye syndrome.
C. exogenous insulin administration.
D. medium chain Acyl CoA dehydrogenase deficiency.
E. glucocorticoid deficiency.

**31. An obese child is likely to have an underlying pathological cause if:**
A. they are tall.
B. their bone age is advanced.
C. they have a scoliosis.
D. they have obese parents.
E. they have hypogonadism.

**32. Regarding growth:**
A. growth velocity accelerates from infancy to puberty.
B. girls begin their adolescent growth spurt on average at age 13.5 years.
C. boys reach maximum height velocity in puberty at around 14 years of age.
D. children reach half their adult height between 2 and 3 years of age.
E. most children with growth hormone deficiency will be detected in the first year of life.

Answers — MCQs in Paediatrics

29. ACD

Lipolysis is one of the main mechanisms for the prevention of hypoglycaemia. Ketones are produced by lipolysis. Insulin inhibits fat breakdown. So any cause of excess insulin will result in non-ketotic hypoglycaemia, as will defects in the pathways of fat metabolism. Ketotic hypoglycaemia implies these pathways are intact but there are other reasons for the hypoglycaemia, such as failure of counter-regulatory hormone response – i.e. cortisol, glucagon and growth hormone deficiency.

30. ABCD

Normal liver function is critical for maintenance of normo-glycaemia. In galactosaemia and Reye syndrome there is pro-gressive liver dysfunction, and this is likely to result in hypoglycaemia. Exogenous insulin will suppress lipolysis and thus result in non-ketotic hypoglycaemia. Medium chain Acyl CoA dehydrogenase is one of the important enzymes of fatty acid oxidation, deficiency of which may result in hypoglycaemia due to failure of fat metabolism. Glucocorticoid deficiency will result in ketotic hypoglycaemia.

31. CE

Overeating causes an increase in growth velocity and such children are usually tall for their age, with an advanced bone age. If, however, there is a pathological cause, the child is likely to be short and fat – e.g. the child with growth hormone deficiency. Genetic and environmental factors are relevant and fat children are more likely to have fat parents. Certain syndromes such as Prader–Willi and Laurence–Moon–Biedl are associated with an insatiable appetite, as well as other features such as scoliosis and hypogonadism.

32. CD

Growth decelerates from infancy to puberty, accelerates through the initial pubertal growth spurt, decelerates then stops once the bones are fused. In girls the growth spurt starts at the onset of pubertal development, but in boys starts half-way through puberty. Surprisingly, most children reach half their final adult height around 2.5 years. For the first 1–2 years of life growth is largely dependent on nutrition, and after that time growth is dependent on hormonal control, so growth hormone deficiency often goes undetected for the first year or two of life.

33. **Regarding puberty:**
    A. girls start pubertal development on average 2 years before boys.
    B. the first indication of pubertal development in boys is facial hair.
    C. the male pubertal growth spurt starts in mid-puberty with 3–4 ml testes.
    D. the female pubertal growth spurt starts at the onset of puberty.
    E. in girls the onset of menstruation occurs in mid-puberty.

34. **Causes of precocious puberty are:**
    A. raised intracranial pressure.
    B. Turner syndrome.
    C. panhypopituitarism.
    D. primary hypothyroidism.
    E. congenital adrenal hypoplasia.

35. **The clinical features of Turner syndrome include:**
    A. tall stature.
    B. polydactyly.
    C. ovarian failure.
    D. hydrocephalus.
    E. asplenism.

**33.  D**

Girls enter puberty earlier than boys – at 10.5 years compared to 11.5 years. The first indication of pubertal development in boys is testicular enlargement; in girls it is development of the breast bud. The female growth spurt starts at the onset of puberty, the male growth spurt in mid-puberty – i.e. at 8–10 ml size testes. The onset of menses is the final event in female pubertal development.

**34.  AD**

Puberty is defined as precocious when development occurs before the age of 8 years in girls and 9 years in boys. In 90% of girls a pathological cause is not found, and the converse is true for boys. All children with precocious puberty should be investigated. Raised intracranial pressure may present with central precocious puberty due to activation of the gonado-trophin axis. Hypothyroidism can present with delayed and precocious puberty – high thyrotrophin-releasing hormone levels can also stimulate prolactin and gonadotrophin release. Ovarian dysgenesis and failure is a feature of Turner syndrome. Panhypopituitarism results in pubertal failure with lack of gonadotrophin production. Congenital adrenal hypoplasia will not cause precocious puberty – adrenal androgens produce virilisation but not enlargement of the gonads.

**35.  C**

The features of Turner syndrome include short stature, neonatal lymphoedema, broad chest with widely spaced nipples, webbed neck, low posterior hair line, high arched palate, wide carrying angle, short 4th and 5th metacarpals, hypoplastic or malformed nails, cardiac and renal abnormal-ities. However, the physical manifestations are variable.

# 18

# Dermatology

1. **Regarding the skin:**
   A. the skin accounts for 15% of total body weight.
   B. the dermis is the main barrier in the skin to fluid and electrolyte loss.
   C. melanocytes distribute melanin through the basal layer of the epidermis.
   D. the dermis is composed mainly of adipose tissue.
   E. temperature regulation is under autonomic control within the epidermis.

2. **Regarding topical treatments for skin conditions:**
   A. lotions are used for exudative rashes.
   B. ointments have a greasy base and should be used for dry skin conditions.
   C. creams are oil and water emulsions.
   D. ointments are not topically absorbed.
   E. creams do not contain any preservative.

3. **Congenital melanocytic naevi:**
   A. are present at birth.
   B. have an irregular margin with long dark hairs.
   C. are associated with leptomeningeal involvement when present on the head.
   D. do not undergo malignant change.
   E. increase in size in proportion to the patient's growth.

4. **Acquired melanocytic naevi:**
   A. appear during the first 6 months of life.
   B. commence as brown or black macules.
   C. are due to a clustering of naevus cells at the dermo-epidermal junction.
   D. have undergone malignant change if surrounded by a depigmented halo.
   E. the risk of malignant change is greater in acquired than congenital naevi.

1. **AC**

   The skin is a complex organ with many functions. It accounts for approximately 15% of body weight. It is composed of three layers: the epidermis, the dermis and the subcutis. The horny layer on the external surface of the epidermis is the main barrier to fluid and electrolyte loss. Protection against UV light is by melanin secreted from the melanocytes in the epidermis. Temperature regulation, via the superficial and deep plexuses in the dermis, is under autonomic control. The subcutis consists mainly of adipose tissue which acts as insulation.

2. **ABC**

   The type of vehicle used depends on the skin problem. Certain preparations are much better tolerated by patients. Creams are generally preferred but are not as useful for dry skin conditions. They are often used as a transport for steroids. Significant systemic absorption may be achieved both with creams and ointments. Creams may contain antimicrobial preservatives which may exacerbate some skin conditions.

3. **ABCE**

   They are present at birth and are classified as large (>20 cm), medium (1.5–20 cm) and small (<1.5 cm). They occur as raised lesions, varying shades of brown to black, with irregular margins and dark hairs. If present over the head or neck, they are associated with leptomeningeal involvement. There is a definite risk of malignant change, usually to melanoma. The lesions at greatest risk of malignant change are the largest, which may be impossible to remove.

4. **BC**

   They appear after the 1st year of life, as brown or black macules. They are due to a clustering of naevus cells at the dermo-epidermal junction, some with intradermal naevus component. Halo naevi due to depigmentation around the lesion are benign. Acquired melanocytic naevi have a low risk of malignant change (less than 0.1%), compared to approximately 5% for congenital naevi.

5. **Strawberry haemangiomas:**
   A. are present from birth.
   B. grow rapidly over the first 6 months.
   C. are lobulated, bright red tumours.
   D. involute with the appearance of grey areas.
   E. disappear in 90% of cases by 9 years.

6. **Complications of haemangiomas include:**
   A. delayed dentition.
   B. ulceration.
   C. amblyopia.
   D. thrombocytopenia.
   E. tracheal compression.

7. **Telangiectatic naevi are the typical lesion in the following conditions:**
   A. 'salmon patch' or 'stork mark'.
   B. port wine stain.
   C. cavernous haemangioma.
   D. Sturge–Weber syndrome.
   E. tuberose sclerosis.

8. **A child with hypohydrotic ectodermal dysplasia will:**
   A. have hypertrichosis.
   B. be at risk of hyperthermia due to hypohidrosis.
   C. suffer recurrent chest infections.
   D. have inherited the syndrome as X-linked recessive.
   E. have dry eyes.

5.  **BCDE**

    Strawberry haemangiomas are usually not present at birth, but develop over the first few weeks of life. The lesion then rapidly grows into a lobulated, well-demarcated, bright red tumour. The rapid growth continues over the first 6 months; the growth rate then slows, and after a stationary phase, involution occurs. The tumour becomes softer and less bulky.

6.  **BCDE**

    Ulceration may occur during the period of rapid growth. If secondary infection is controlled, the ulcer usually heals within a few weeks often with some scarring. Amblyopia may occur if the lesion closes the eye even for 4 weeks in infancy. Large cavernous haemangiomas are occasionally associated with the Kasabach–Merritt syndrome when thrombocytopenia is caused by entrapment of platelets within the lesion. There may be a consumptive coagulopathy. Lesions involving the upper airway may cause respiratory compromise.

7.  **ABD**

    The salmon patch is a group of dilated dermal capillaries present at birth in up to 50% of infants. The classical 'stork mark' occurs on the nape of the neck, brow, upper eyelids or upper lip. Almost all facial lesions fade by 1 year, but lesions at the nape of the neck may persist. A port wine stain is a vascular malformation composed of dilated mature capillaries and is present from birth as a deep pink colour in infancy, later becoming purple. Sturge–Weber syndrome is the association of a facial port wine stain and a vascular malformation of the ipsilateral meninges. The skin lesions in tuberose sclerosis are depigmented naevi.

8.  **BCDE**

    The primary defect in hypohydrotic ectodermal dysplasia is in tissue of ectodermal origin, with a combination of teeth, hair, sweat gland, skin, eye and mucosal abnormalities. The hair is sparse, fine and fair. Absence of sweat glands may cause hyperthermia when the ambient temperature rises. Thick respiratory tract secretions predispose to infection. Hypoplasia of the nasolacrimal ducts causes dry eyes.

9. **The cutaneous manifestations of tuberous sclerosis include:**
   A. dermatitis herpetiformis.
   B. angiofibromas.
   C. periungual fibromas.
   D. café au lait patches.
   E. aplasia cutis.

10. **The diagnosis of neurofibromatosis is often made on the cutaneous manifestations of the disease. They include:**
    A. linear groups of vesicles.
    B. erythematous plaques with thick, silvery white scale.
    C. a minimum of 20 café au lait macules greater than 5 cm in diameter.
    D. small freckle-like pigmented macules in the axillae.
    E. cutaneous neurofibroma.

11. **Regarding Herpes simplex virus (HSV) infection in children:**
    A. serological studies show >90% of the population have been infected by adulthood.
    B. neonatal HSV infection presents in a dermatomal distribution.
    C. primary herpetic gingivostomatitis progresses to systemic HSV infection in >75% of cases.
    D. disseminated HSV infection occurs as a complication of atopic eczema.
    E. 50% of HSV infection is due to HSV II.

12. **Herpes zoster infection (shingles):**
    A. is not infectious.
    B. occurs in a bilateral dermatomal distribution.
    C. if present before the age of 1 year, it indicates maternal chickenpox during the pregnancy.
    D. involving the trigeminal nerve causes keratitis and uveitis.
    E. in a child indicates an underlying immunological deficiency or malignancy.

### 9. BC

Tuberous sclerosis is one of the neurocutaneous disorders. The pathognomonic features are: angiofibromas – papules in a butterfly distribution over the bridge of the nose; periungual fibromas – firm, smooth flesh-coloured papules; shagreen patches – a connective tissue naevus; and ash leaf macules – depigmented macules. Café au lait patches are no more common than in the general population.

### 10. DE

The café au lait macule is the commonest feature of NF type 1 and the diagnostic criteria include: at least six macules of at least 1.5 cm in diameter. In 20% of cases, small freckle-like macules occur in the axillae. Cutaneous neurofibroma are soft, pink sessile or pedunculated tumours that usually appear after puberty.

### 11. AD

Herpes simplex virus infection is common and the primary infection may be asymptomatic. More than 90% of the population have been infected by adulthood. Neonatal HSV infection usually results from transfer from the mother's vagina during delivery, without treatment with antivirals disseminated infection is typical. After the perinatal period, a primary infection may present as a herpetic stomatitis with lesions in the mouth and on the lips. Stomatitis infection does not usually disseminate and antivirals are not indicated in an otherwise healthy child. HSV I may disseminate in atopic eczema (eczema herpeticum) due to the associated T-cell defect. The majority of infections are due to HSV I; HSV II is the infectious agent in genital herpes.

### 12. CD

Herpes zoster infection is due to reactivation of the zoster virus, from the dorsal root or cranial nerve ganglia. It does not commonly occur in children, but it is not indicative of underlying pathology. The lesions occur in a unilateral dermatome distribution and the vesicles do shed the virus, so transmission of infection is possible. If the infection involves the ophthalmic division of the trigeminal nerve, the possibility of eye involvement (keratitis and uveitis) necessitates treatment with anti-viral agents. Shingles in a child less than 1 year old indicates transplacental infection.

13. **Molluscum contagiosum:**
    A. are caused by the pox virus.
    B. are white lesions with a central umbilication.
    C. resolve spontaneously within 4–6 months.
    D. are due to viral activation from the dorsal root ganglia.
    E. are treated with oral acyclovir.

14. **Children with atopic eczema:**
    A. have an increased tendency to form IgE antibodies to inhalants and foods.
    B. do not have an increased susceptibility to asthma.
    C. show signs of eczema prior to 6 months of age in more than 75% of cases.
    D. have a tendency to lichenification of their skin.
    E. do not have facial involvement.

15. **Patients with atopic eczema are at increased risk of:**
    A. Molluscum contagiosum.
    B. widespread Herpes simplex infection.
    C. impetigo.
    D. severe erythema multiforme (Stevens–Johnson syndrome).
    E. alopecia.

16. **The following may produce a rash involving the perineal area:**
    A. candidal infection.
    B. ammoniacal contact.
    C. seborrhoeic dermatitis.
    D. laundering products.
    E. zinc deficiency.

**13. ABC**

Molluscum contagiosum are caused by the pox virus and are common in children aged 1–4 years. Spread is by close contact. The lesions may be numerous; they are pearly white, raised lesions with a central umbilication, size varying from 1 to 10 mm in diameter. They resolve spontaneously without treatment in 4–6 months. Oral acyclovir is of no benefit.

**14. ACD**

Atopy is a genetically determined disorder, with an increased tendency to form IgE antibodies to inhalants and foods. They have an increased susceptibility to asthma, allergic rhinitis and eczema. The characteristic clinical features of atopic eczema are a generalised dryness and tendency to lichenification of the skin. The eczema may begin at any age but 75% of patients show the first signs before 6 months. The predominant area affected in infants is the face, progressing to limb flexures in the older child.

**15. ABC**

Pruritis and excoriation are typical of atopic eczema. The risk of infection with bacteria and viruses is greater than for the child with intact skin. They are not at greater risk of erythema multiforme, an immune complex mediated vasculitis that typically follows certain infections.

**16. ABCDE**

Napkin dermatitis is the term applied when the skin of the nappy area is involved. Urine is the primary irritant (ammonia from urine is irritant) and moist skin is easily infected with candida. Seborrhoeic dermatitis may only involve the nappy area, although classically the rash also involves the scalp (known as cradle cap), the ears, the nasolabial folds and axillae. Allergy to laundering products may cause a dermatitis. In zinc deficiency there is a rash known as acrodermatitis enteropathica which may be perioral and perianal. Diarrhoea and alopecia are also features. There is defective absorption of zinc – all the features rapidly disappear when high doses of zinc are administered.

**17. Vesicular lesions are typical in:**
   **A.** Henoch Schönlein purpura.
   **B.** vitiligo.
   **C.** Herpes simplex infection.
   **D.** systemic lupus erythematosus.
   **E.** Varicella zoster infection.

**17.  CE**

Vesicles are fluid-filled blisters – culture of the fluid may reveal an infectious agent. Typically chickenpox (Varicella zoster infection) and Herpes simplex are vesicular eruptions. Henoch-Schönlein purpura is a vasculitic lesion. Vitiligo may be an autoimmune disease causing depigmentation of the skin. SLE typically presents with an erythematous butterfly rash on the face.

# 19

## Cardiology

1. **Congenital heart disease may present with:**
   A. failure to thrive.
   B. recurrent vomiting.
   C. excessive sweating.
   D. an asymptomatic murmur in a 15-year-old.
   E. cyanosis becoming apparent 2 days after birth.

2. **The following clinical findings are correctly paired with the relevant cardiac lesion:**
   A. upper limb hypertension in patent ductus arteriosus.
   B. single second heart sound in atrial septal defect.
   C. an ejection click in aortic stenosis.
   D. a loud second heart sound in pulmonary hypertension.
   E. a pansystolic murmur in atrial septal defect.

3. **The following clinical findings are supportive of a diagnosis of heart failure in an infant:**
   A. inability to complete a normal feed.
   B. a heart rate of 180 beats per minute at rest.
   C. facial oedema.
   D. hepatomegaly.
   E. a chest radiograph showing reduced pulmonary vascular markings.

4. **The following therapeutic interventions are likely to be beneficial:**
   A. frusemide for a child with a large ventricular septal defect.
   B. amiloride for a patient on high-dose diuretic therapy.
   C. supplementary oxygen in transposition of the great arteries.
   D. surgical closure of a patent foramen ovale.
   E. prostaglandin E1 therapy in transposition of the great arteries.

1. **ACDE**

   Congenital heart disease presents with a murmur, cyanosis or signs of heart failure – singly or in combination. Heart failure causes sweating due to increased sympathetic drive. Vomiting is due to bowel and hepatic congestion, but is unlikely to be a presenting symptom. Increased calorie requirements and poor intake result in poor weight gain. In cyanotic lesions, such as pulmonary atresia or where there is mixing of the systemic and pulmonary circulations (transposition), closure of the ductus arteriosus causes cyanosis. An atrial septal defect may present as an asymptomatic murmur at any age.

2. **CD**

   Upper limb hypertension occurs in coarctation of the aorta. In an atrial septal defect there is characteristically fixed splitting of the second sound and a soft ejection systolic murmur, whereas the normal aortic and pulmonary sounds come together in expiration. An ejection click is an additional sound in early systole which may occur in aortic or pulmonary valve stenosis.

3. **ABCD**

   Infants with cardiac failure (most commonly due to a large left to right shunt) present with tachypnoea (secondary to pulmonary congestion) and tachycardia. Breathlessness in infants may be reported by parents as difficulty in completing a feed. Ankle oedema is not characteristic of heart failure in infancy, more commonly liver enlargement and facial puffiness occur. Pulmonary congestion produces increased vascular markings on the chest radiograph.

4. **ABE**

   Diuretic therapy is beneficial where a left to right shunt (e.g. a VSD) causes heart failure. Loop diuretics commonly cause hypokalaemia and are often used in combination with potassium supplements or potassium-sparing diuretics. Oxygen therapy is rarely of benefit in cyanotic conditions. The foramen ovale is a defect in the atrial septum, which usually closes soon after birth but often remains patent for some months. It is asymptomatic. In cyanotic conditions presenting soon after birth, an infusion of prostaglandin re-opens the arterial duct, which will improve systemic oxygenation.

5. **When investigating congenital heart disease:**
   A. electrocardiography and chest radiology can provide a definitive diagnosis in most cases.
   B. electrocardiographic criteria for diagnosing ventricular hypertrophy are the same as those employed in adults.
   C. cardiac catheterisation remains necessary in the majority of cases.
   D. Doppler echocardiography can provide an estimate of the pressure gradient across a stenotic valve.
   E. cardiac catheterisation is required if accurate measurement of a left to right shunt is required.

6. **Major criteria for the diagnosis of rheumatic fever include:**
   A. choreiform limb movements.
   B. migratory polyarthritis.
   C. a soft ejection systolic murmur at the left sternal edge.
   D. an elevated ESR.
   E. a previous history of rheumatic fever.

7. **Regarding infectious endocarditis:**
   A. most cases occur in structurally normal hearts.
   B. diagnosis is often delayed because of the non-specific symptoms.
   C. echocardiography can be helpful in supporting the diagnosis.
   D. treatment with 10 days of intravenous antibiotic is generally sufficient.
   E. antibiotic treatment for 5 days following a surgical procedure is necessary to reduce the risk of endocarditis in vulnerable patients.

8. **The following findings are compatible with a diagnosis of innocent murmur:**
   A. variation in the loudness of the murmur with a change in posture.
   B. a murmur heard in early diastole.
   C. a thrill.
   D. an ejection click.
   E. a continuous murmur.

5. **DE**

   Although clinical features, chest radiology and electrocardiography can sometimes provide a definitive diagnosis, many cases of congenital heart disease require further imaging to identify the lesion correctly. Normal values for the ECG vary with age and differ from adults. Echocardiography is used to assess the anatomical abnormality. Cardiac echo with Doppler studies has reduced the need for cardiac catheterisation, which may still be necessary if accurate assessment of pressure gradients, shunts or pulmonary hypertension is required.

6. **AB**

   Criteria for the diagnosis of rheumatic fever include evidence of recent Streptococcal infection, as well as two major criteria, or alternatively, one major and two minor criteria. In addition to those given in the question, major criteria include evidence of carditis (tachycardia, heart failure, the development of new murmurs), erythema marginatum and the development of nodules over bony prominences. Minor criteria are fever, arthralgia, previous history of rheumatic fever, raised ESR or C-reactive protein and prolonged PR interval on the electrocardiogram.

7. **BC**

   Endocarditis is rare in children with normal hearts. The symptoms are often insidious and include lethargy, anorexia and intermittent fever. Diagnosis requires the identification of the organism by blood culture but echocardiography showing intracardiac vegetations would be supportive of the diagnosis. Endocarditis can prove difficult to eliminate and may require 6 weeks of antibiotic treatment. 24 hours' antibiotic treatment perioperative period provides effective prophylaxis for at-risk patients.

8. **AE**

   Innocent heart murmurs are common. There are various types, but they are characteristically systolic, are soft or have a 'musical' quality, and are heard along the left sternal edge or at the root of the neck. A venous hum is a continuous murmur which is heard over the sterno-clavicular joints and may disappear when the patient lies down. Innocent murmurs are never diastolic, never associated with a thrill and abnormalities of the heart sounds are not found.

9. **The following are examples of cyanotic congenital heart defects:**
   A. tetralogy of Fallot.
   B. transposition of the great arteries.
   C. patent arterial duct.
   D. coarctation of the aorta.
   E. tricuspid atresia.

10. **Ventricular septal defects:**
    A. may present as asymptomatic murmurs.
    B. are commonly associated with a thrill.
    C. which cause heart failure will require surgical closure in more than 90% of cases.
    D. generally require cardiac catheterisation to make a confident diagnosis.
    E. with pulmonary hypertension are fatal if not corrected.

11. **In a child with an atrial septal defect (ostium secundum defect):**
    A. there is likely to be a systolic murmur due to mitral regurgitation.
    B. major limitation of exercise tolerance is likely.
    C. cardiac catheterisation is unlikely to be necessary.
    D. closure should be performed by the age of 2 years at the latest.
    E. the surgical mortality is around 10%.

12. **Persistent ductus arteriosus:**
    A. connects the pulmonary artery and descending aorta.
    B. is a problem confined to premature infants.
    C. causes a continuous 'machinery' murmur.
    D. only requires closure if symptomatic.
    E. is likely to close in response to indomethicin in a 2-year-old child.

9.  **ABE**

    Congenital heart lesions cause cyanosis by reducing pulmonary blood flow (e.g. tetralogy of Fallot, tricuspid atresia), by causing extensive mixing of de-oxygenated blood with oxygenated (e.g. truncus arteriosus, 'single ventricle' malformations) or by preventing the pulmonary venous drainage reaching the systemic circulation (e.g. transposition of the great arteries). In many cases, two of these mechanisms may be operating. In patent arterial duct there is increased pulmonary blood flow. Coarctation causes heart failure, but not cyanosis until late.

10. **ABCE**

    Ventricular septal defect (VSD) is the commonest congenital cardiac defect. Many are small, asymptomatic and only identified by detecting a murmur during physical examination. These small defects will often close spontaneously. Large defects cause heart failure after the 1st month of life. Moderate defects may not cause major symptoms, but may lead to pulmonary hypertension. The diagnosis of VSD is generally confirmed by echocardiography.

11. **C**

    Atrial septal defect is usually asymptomatic and is detected by finding a systolic murmur during examination. The murmur is due to increased blood flow across the pulmonary valve. The diagnosis is confirmed by echocardiography. Atrial septal defects are generally closed surgically or by interventional catheterisation before school age. In experienced hands, the mortality is less than 1%. Pulmonary vascular disease does not develop as rapidly as with a large ventricular septal defect.

12. **AC**

    In utero the ductus arteriosus diverts blood from the lungs. The duct normally closes soon after birth. Persistence of the duct is commonly but not exclusively found in premature infants. The flow of blood from aorta to pulmonary artery causes a continuous murmur extending through systole and into diastole. Prostaglandins play a role in maintaining duct patency, and indomethacin is effective in closing the ductus in premature infants but ineffective in older children. Surgery is always indicated because the risk of endocarditis exceeds the risk of surgery.

13. **Coarctation of the aorta may present with:**
    A. clinical features suggestive of septic shock in an infant.
    B. an asymptomatic murmur.
    C. pain in the legs on exercise in a school-age child.
    D. rib notching on a chest X-ray.
    E. postural hypotension in an adolescent.

14. **Aortic stenosis:**
    A. is associated with Noonan syndrome.
    B. is unlikely to occur in the presence of a bicuspid aortic valve.
    C. usually presents with symptoms before school age.
    D. can be treated by trans-catheter balloon valvuloplasty.
    E. will not require treatment if asymptomatic.

15. **Pulmonary stenosis:**
    A. is an uncommon cardiac lesion in childhood.
    B. usually presents with symptoms before school age.
    C. causes an ejection systolic murmur at the left sternal edge.
    D. in severe cases, causes right ventricular hypertrophic changes on ECG.
    E. can often be treated by balloon valvuloplasty at cardiac catheterisation.

16. **Following the birth of an infant with transposition of the great arteries:**
    A. features of shock are likely to develop within minutes of birth.
    B. the defect is difficult to diagnose without performing cardiac catheterisation.
    C. balloon septostomy will increase mixing between right and left ventricles.
    D. maintenance of adequate oxygenation is dependent on mixing via the foramen ovale and arterial duct.
    E. the 'switch' operation should result in a complete anatomical correction.

**13.   ABCD**

Coarctation of the aorta presenting in infancy causes profound, acute, circulatory failure. Septic shock is an important differential diagnosis. Less severely affected individuals may present later in life with upper limb hypertension, or some children describe pain in the legs on exercise due to diminished lower limb blood flow. The obstruction to the thoracic aorta results in blood diversion along intercostal vessels which become dilated and may cause rib notching.

**14.   D**

Aortic stenosis and coarctation is associated with Turner syndrome, and pulmonary stenosis with Noonan syndrome. Aortic valve stenosis commonly occurs when there is a congenitally malformed bicuspid valve. A minority of cases with very severe stenosis present with circulatory failure in the neonatal period, termed critical aortic stenosis. The majority of cases are asymptomatic through childhood and are diagnosed by the finding of an asymptomatic murmur. Treatment may be by balloon or surgical valvuloplasty or valve replacement. Treatment is indicated for relief of symptoms or a pressure gradient indicating severe stenosis.

**15.   CDE**

Pulmonary stenosis is the commonest obstructive cardiac lesion in childhood. The great majority of cases are mild and are often non-progressive. Symptoms are uncommon. When there is a significant stenosis, treatment has generally been by surgical valvuloplasty but, in recent years, many have successfully been treated by balloon valvuloplasty.

**16.   DE**

In transposition of the great arteries there are two separate circulations: one perfusing the lungs, and the other the systemic circulation. Oxygenated blood must reach the systemic circulation through the foramen ovale, the arterial duct or, in some cases, through a ventricular septal defect. Prostaglandins are used to keep the duct open and a septostomy is performed to enlarge the communication between the atria. The diagnosis is established by echocardiography. The 'switch' operation repositions the great arteries in the correct locations.

17. **In tetralogy of Fallot:**
    A. cyanosis is usually clinically apparent within a few days of birth.
    B. cyanosis is typically increased during crying.
    C. creation of a systemic to pulmonary shunt is rarely beneficial.
    D. beta blockers are ineffective in preventing cyanotic episodes.
    E. children typically 'squat' following exertion.

18. **A child with supraventricular tachycardia:**
    A. probably has structural congenital heart disease.
    B. is likely to collapse soon after the onset of symptoms.
    C. is likely to respond to intravenous adenosine.
    D. should not be treated with DC cardioversion.
    E. is likely to have a prolonged PR interval on resting ECG.

19. **Regarding atrioventricular septal defects:**
    A. abnormalities of mitral and tricuspid valves are to be expected.
    B. clinical symptoms are usually apparent in the neonatal period.
    C. surgical repair is needed early if there is evidence of pulmonary hypertension.
    D. defects in the atrial septum are typically found 'high' in the septum.
    E. the lesion is more common in children with Down syndrome.

20. **In tricuspid atresia:**
    A. systemic venous return passes exclusively through the foramen ovale.
    B. pulmonary perfusion depends on a patent duct or ventricular septal defect.
    C. the commonest presentation is with cyanosis at a few weeks of age.
    D. a systemic to pulmonary shunt is likely to be needed in the short term.
    E. 'corrective' surgery redirects the systemic venous return directly into the pulmonary circulation.

**17.  BE**

Severe cases of tetralogy of Fallot present with cyanosis in the newborn period, but most affected babies do not become cyanosed until several months of age due to increasing right ventricular outflow tract obstruction. Spells of cyanosis occur during exertion and with crying. Beta blockers are effective in preventing these episodes. Affected children typically 'squat', which probably increases venous return and increases systemic vascular resistance, both of which increase blood flow to the pulmonary artery. For persistent cyanosis surgery is required, either palliative (systemic to pulmonary shunt) or corrective, depending on the age of the child and the surgical prospects.

**18.  C**

Supraventricular tachycardia usually occurs in children with structurally normal hearts. There is often an accessory pathway between atria and ventricles which can be detected by identifying an abnormally short PR interval on ECG. Supraventricular tachycardia is tolerated by children surprisingly well; drug therapy is the treatment of choice. A minority of patients develop circulatory failure, and in these cases, DC cardioversion is indicated.

**19.  ACE**

Atrioventricular septal defects (AVSDs) involve tissue adjacent to the mitral and tricuspid valves. The lesion therefore comprises various defects of lower atrial septum, upper ventricular septum and the atrioventricular valves leaflets which may be 'cleft' and incompetent. Symptoms rarely present in the neonatal period, but more commonly at between 2 and 12 months. Surgical repair of the valves can be difficult and is often deferred to allow the child to grow, but if there is evidence of pulmonary hypertension, surgical intervention is planned earlier.

**20.  ABCDE**

Despite the abnormal anatomy, it is common for these children to be discharged home and to present a few weeks later with cyanosis or another symptom. At that time, pulmonary perfusion can be augmented by a systemic to pulmonary shunt, but in the long term, an adequate pulmonary circulation depends on the creation of an anastomosis between systemic return and pulmonary artery (the Fontan procedure).

# 20

## Paediatric accident and emergency medicine and intensive care

1. **Between 1 and 14 years of age:**
   A. the commonest cause of death is trauma.
   B. less than 1% of deaths can be attributed to congenital abnormalities.
   C. malignant disease accounts for 10–20% of deaths.
   D. the importance of infection as a primary cause of death declines with increasing age.
   E. sudden infant death syndrome is responsible for around 5% of deaths.

2. **When resuscitating a child:**
   A. the neck should be fully extended to open the airway.
   B. who is asystolic, cardiac massage should be initiated before ventilation.
   C. electrical defibrillation is rarely indicated.
   D. an intraosseous needle is a useful means of gaining access to the circulation.
   E. if there has been no cardiac output for 20 min, the prognosis is better than for an adult in a comparable situation.

3. **The following drugs can be given to a child through an endotracheal tube:**
   A. adrenaline.
   B. calcium gluconate.
   C. sodium bicarbonate.
   D. lignocaine.
   E. atropine.

4. **Regarding resuscitation of a child:**
   A. bag and mask ventilation is unlikely to be effective.
   B. the inspired oxygen concentration should be maintained below 40%.
   C. the correct size of endotracheal tube can be estimated from the child's age.
   D. external cardiac massage has to be performed very gently to prevent rib fractures.
   E. defibrillator output is adjusted according to estimated weight.

1. **ACD**

   Major causes of death before 1 year are premature birth, congenital abnormalities and sudden infant death syndrome (SIDS). By definition, SIDS cannot occur after 1 year of age. After 1 year, the commonest causes of death in children are trauma, congenital abnormalities and malignant disease in that order. Maturation of the immune system and immunisation mean that infection becomes progressively less important as a cause of death with advancing age.

2. **CD**

   Resuscitation of a child follows the same principles employed for an adult: airway, breathing and circulation – 'ABC'. The chin is gently extended, so that the nose is 'sniffing the air', but not fully extended. Even if the patient is asystolic, ventilation should be established before cardiac massage since there is no point in pumping deoxygenated blood around the body. Unlike adults, where myocardial disease is an important cause of cardiorespiratory arrest, loss of cardiac activity in children generally occurs as a late event in a process which began with respiratory failure or hypotension. For this reason, the prognosis in children with asystole is worse than in their adult counterparts. Ventricular fibrillation is an uncommon arrythmia in children and defibrillation is required infrequently. An intraosseous needle, inserted into the marrow cavity below and medial to the tibial tuberosity, gives rapid access to the circulation in collapsed children when intravenous access is difficult.

3. **ADE**

   The endotracheal route is useful for administering drugs while establishing vascular access.

4. **CE**

   Bag and mask ventilation is often highly effective. Unrestricted oxygen can be hazardous in preterm infants and in adults with chronic respiratory failure; such restrictions do not apply to children. As in other areas of paediatrics, account must be taken of the child's size; simple formulae exist for calculation of drug doses, size of endotracheal tube and correct defibrillator output.

5. **Burns in children:**
   A. occur equally across all social classes.
   B. which occur within the house most commonly happen in the kitchen.
   C. cannot be caused by ordinary household bathwater.
   D. are regularly caused by unrestricted exposure to the sun.
   E. could have been prevented in the majority of cases.

6. **The following features should raise serious suspicion of physical abuse:**
   A. a skull fracture in a 6-week-old baby who allegedly rolled off the bed.
   B. a torn lingual frenulum in a 2-year-old.
   C. bruises of various ages over the shins in a 6-year-old.
   D. bruises of various ages over the back and buttocks in a 6-year-old.
   E. a report by an 8-year-old sibling of excessive beating.

7. **When a doctor suspects that a child may have been the victim of physical abuse:**
   A. the physical examination should be extremely limited so as not to arouse the parents' suspicion.
   B. particular care is needed to make an accurate record of any injuries.
   C. information about whether or not the child's name is on the 'At-risk Register' will be helpful.
   D. the parents should always be confronted with the allegation of child abuse immediately.
   E. an Emergency Protection Order should always be obtained to remove the child from further risk.

8. **The following are associated with non-accidental injury:**
   A. a changing account of how the injury occurred.
   B. retinal haemorrhages.
   C. rushing to obtain medical attention for a trivial injury.
   D. demanding a second opinion.
   E. a prolonged prothrombin time.

5.  **BDE**

    Children from socio-economically disadvantaged homes are at increased risk of burns. Accidental burns are most often due to spilling of hot liquids. In many homes tap water is sufficiently hot to scald. Every summer, A&E departments deal with severe cases of sunburn, some of which require hospital admission.

6.  **ABDE**

    When a child is brought to hospital with an injury, a number of features may raise suspicion of abuse. These include injuries incompatible with the child's age (6-week-old babies cannot roll over), injuries in unusual places and a direct allegation of abuse by the child, a sibling or another adult.

7.  **BC**

    When physical abuse is suspected, it is always particularly important to make a full physical examination for other evidence of injury or physical illness and to make a careful record of the findings. Medical notes may be required as legal evidence many months later when the doctor will have difficulty remembering precise details. Sensitivity and flexibility is needed in dealing with each case. The allegation of child abuse is distressing and cannot be made without significant evidence. Consultation with a senior colleague is essential. Legal measures for ensuring a child's safety should be restricted to cases where there is evidence of continuing risk. If parental cooperation can be secured, this is preferable. The 'At-risk Register' is a file containing names of children living in the area about whom there has been concern because of previous incidents.

8.  **AB**

    An inconsistent or variable history of an injury and delay in seeking medical attention indicate that an injury may not be accidental. Anxious or concerned parents may prove difficult to deal with, but parents who have injured their child are unlikely to want to draw attention to themselves. Physical disorders which can cause bruising or fractures need to be considered.

9. **When evaluating a 5-year-old who may have been sexually abused:**
   A. questions about sexual practices need to be asked repeatedly.
   B. the child may feel she is betraying her family by disclosure.
   C. genital examination should be performed urgently.
   D. abnormal physical findings are present in most cases of sexual abuse.
   E. it is important to recognise that the perpetrator is most likely to be an adult outside the child's immediate family circle.

10. **When resuscitating a child following a near-drowning accident:**
   A. the neck should be stabilised as a priority.
   B. there is no value in continuing resuscitation if the core temperature is below 32°C.
   C. peritoneal lavage with warmed dialysate is useful in treating associated hypothermia.
   D. if the child appears lifeless when pulled from the water, there is an extremely poor prognosis.
   E. the response of cardiac arrhythmia to treatment is affected by hypothermia.

11. **In managing an unconscious child:**
   A. identifying the cause of the coma takes precedence over other aspects of care.
   B. endotracheal intubation is contraindicated if there is no gag reflex.
   C. hypoglycaemia is diagnostic of insulin overdose.
   D. ingestion of drugs is an important cause to consider at any age.
   E. a lumbar puncture should be performed promptly.

12. **The following interventions can be useful if there is raised intracranial pressure:**
   A. elevating the head of the bed.
   B. adjusting mechanical ventilation to produce a modest rise in arterial $CO_2$.
   C. an intravenous infusion of Mannitol.
   D. thiopentone infusion.
   E. restriction of intravenous fluids.

9. **B**

Sexually abused children have often been indoctrinated to believe that disclosure will be damaging to themselves or their family. The child must be asked to recount his or her experiences as spontaneously as possible. Repeated or leading questions can lead to false answers. Urgent examination of the genitalia is rarely required, except in cases where forensic specimens need to be collected, and should always be performed by individuals with expertise in this field. Physical signs may only be present in 10% of sexually abused children. The commonest perpetrator of sexual abuse is a male living in the child's home.

10. **ACE**

Physical injuries are common in this situation and the cervical spine should be stabilised as a priority. Hypothermia slows the metabolic rate and protects against the effects of circulatory arrest. Ventricular fibrillation may be refractory to treatment at low body temperature. Resuscitation should therefore continue until core temperature is at least 32°C. In patients with core temperatures below this level, internal rewarming methods may be necessary. Around 70% of 'lifeless' children will survive if resuscitation is commenced immediately. About 5% of survivors have profound neurological damage.

11. **D**

Priority should always be given to cardiorespiratory status. An absent gag reflex is an indication for endotracheal intubation to prevent aspiration of gastric contents. Hypoglycaemia may be due to endocrine and metabolic disorders and should be excluded since it is readily treatable. Toddlers may ingest drugs left within their reach; older children may take them for 'experimentation' or because of emotional problems. Lumbar puncture is contraindicated in comatose children in case there is raised intracranial pressure.

12. **ACDE**

A low arterial $CO_2$ reduces cerebral blood flow, elevation of the head, modest fluid restriction and administration of Mannitol may reduce cerebral oedema, thiopentone controls seizures and reduces cerebral metabolic rate – all of which may reduce intracranial pressure.

13. **The following are features of iron poisoning:**
    A. gastrointestinal haemorrhage.
    B. circulatory failure.
    C. hepatic failure.
    D. pyloric stenosis.
    E. cerebral oedema.

14. **In a teenager who reports ingesting a large number of paracetamol tablets:**
    A. jaundice is likely to develop within 24 hours.
    B. acetylcysteine must be given within 16 hours in order to be effective.
    C. a prolonged prothrombin time is a marker of impending liver failure.
    D. liver transplantation must be considered if severe hepatic failure develops.
    E. acetylcysteine should be administered irrespective of the paracetamol level.

15. **When dealing with a child who has ingested a toxic substance:**
    A. ipecac is ineffective in emptying the stomach.
    B. gastric lavage is always unhelpful if more than 4 hours have elapsed since the ingestion.
    C. gastric lavage should be performed urgently if the substance taken has corrosive properties.
    D. activated charcoal is likely to be well tolerated.
    E. advice from a Poisons Centre is restricted to overdoses of medication.

16. **Regarding poisoning in children and teenagers:**
    A. most cases of accidental drug ingestion occur between 1 and 3 years of age.
    B. around 5% of cases of accidental drug ingestion are fatal.
    C. the introduction of child-proof containers led to an 85% fall in admissions with accidental ingestion.
    D. 24 hours of observation in hospital is mandatory.
    E. an effective psychiatric evaluation of an adolescent who has taken a drug overdose can be performed in the casualty department.

13. **ABCDE**

Iron preparations are found in many homes and are regularly ingested by young children. As can be seen from the list of complications, iron can be highly toxic in overdose. Pyloric stenosis is a late complication secondary to scarring.

14. **BCD**

Like iron, paracetamol is a widely available drug whose potential for toxicity is not always appreciated. After ingesting the drug, there may be some gastrointestinal upset which is likely to resolve within hours. Clinical signs of hepatic failure present after 2–4 days; early warning of hepatic injury can be obtained by measuring the prothrombin time. In patients with toxic blood levels, hepatic failure can be prevented by giving *N*-acetylcysteine within 16 hours of ingestion. For massive hepatic injury, transplantation is the only option.

15. **None of these – all false**

If the child presents within 4 hours of ingesting a quantity of a substance likely to be toxic, the stomach should be emptied by gastric lavage or by administration of ipecac. Certain drugs (salicylates, tricyclics, antiemetics) delay gastric emptying, in which case emptying the stomach may be worthwhile several hours later. Emptying the stomach by any means is contra-indicated if the substance ingested is corrosive, lipoid or a hydrocarbon. Children may find it impossible to swallow activated charcoal; if necessary, it can be given through a nasogastric tube. Poisons Centres collect data on all varieties of substances which may be ingested, including plants and household products.

16. **AC**

The introduction of child-proof containers was a highly successful child safety measure. Despite the fact that several thousand children present at A&E departments each year, there are less than 20 deaths each year from ingested poisons. Each case must be assessed as potentially serious, but the majority can be discharged home without admission. The presentation of an adolescent following a deliberate drug overdose is common. In general, these patients should be admitted to allow careful consideration of possible severe emotional disturbance or social pressures.

17. **Diabetic ketoacidosis:**
    A. is characteristically associated with slow, irregular respiration.
    B. has a similar presentation to salicylate poisoning.
    C. is almost never the first presentation of diabetes mellitus.
    D. is frequently precipitated by infection.
    E. requires rapid reduction of blood glucose levels to below 15 mmol/L.

18. **Management of a 6-year-old boy with acute asthma should include:**
    A. routine measurement of arterial blood gases on arrival at hospital.
    B. administration of nebulised drugs using compressed air.
    C. continuous nebulised bronchodilator until the condition is stabilised.
    D. chest radiography if there is a poor response to the first 30 min of treatment.
    E. prescription of a mild sedative if the child's anxiety is making treatment difficult.

19. **The following are employed as first- or second-line drugs in the management of status epilepticus:**
    A. rectal diazepam.
    B. intravenous diazepam.
    C. intravenous sodium valproate.
    D. intravenous thiopentone.
    E. rectal paraldehyde.

20. **In a child who has been brought to the casualty department after being hit by a car travelling at 40 miles per hour:**
    A. vascular access is mandatory even if there are no signs of hypovolaemia.
    B. a cervical collar should be applied once cervical radiographs have been obtained.
    C. hypotension requires immediate infusion of an inotropic drug.
    D. replacement of blood should await fully cross-matched blood.
    E. full assessment of injuries should be deferred until airway, breathing and circulation have been stabilised.

17.  **BD**

Diabetic ketoacidosis is a common presentation for new cases. Insulin deficiency leads to ketone production and metabolic acidosis which, in turn, causes hyperventilation. Initially, the clinical features may appear similar to salicylate poisoning or renal failure, but basic biochemical investigation will establish the diagnosis. The aim is to correct the hyperglycaemia gradually (over 48 hours) since rapid changes in osmolarity can aggravate cerebral oedema.

18.  **CD**

Arterial blood gases are best deferred until essential for management. Pulse oximetry with capillary gases provides a good estimate of oxygenation, pH and $PCO_2$. Nebulisers should be driven by oxygen to prevent hypoxia. In severe acute asthma nebulised bronchodilators may be given continuously, unless there is evidence of adverse effects such as severe tremulousness, hypokalaemia or extreme tachycardia. In most cases, the chest X-ray does not alter management, but one should be obtained if there is a poor clinical response to therapy. Sedation is inadvisable in any patient at risk of respiratory failure.

19.  **ABE**

In acute epilepsy venous access may be difficult and some drugs can be administered rectally. Clinical practice may vary, but in general, diazepam and/or paraldehyde are administered first, followed by phenytoin or phenobarbitone if necessary. Thiopentone is employed with muscle relaxant and mechanical ventilation in persistent seizures when other measures have failed.

20.  **AE**

Stabilisation of cardiorespiratory status and of spinal alignment take precedence over other injuries. A cervical collar should be applied as soon as possible; a spinal injury should be assumed until proven otherwise. Vasoconstriction may compensate for hypovolaemia and severe hypotension may develop only at a relatively late stage. Any child with significant trauma should have secure vascular access as a routine. Hypotension in this setting is almost certainly due to blood loss even if the source of haemorrhage is not evident; circulating volume should be restored promptly with colloid, crystalloid or O-negative blood.

21. **When managing a child with a serious head injury:**
    A. priority should be given to assessment and management of the airway, breathing and circulation.
    B. the greater the force of the injury, the greater the risk of brain damage.
    C. CT scan of the head is mandatory if the Glasgow Coma Score is 5 or less.
    D. by the time the child reaches hospital, medical treatment cannot affect the severity of brain damage.
    E. the extent of external head injury does not relate to the severity of brain damage.

22. **In the management of a child with hyperkalaemia:**
    A. a serum potassium of 6.0 mmol/L causes a high risk of cardiac arrythmia.
    B. intravenous calcium is contraindicated if an arrhythmia is present.
    C. intravenous salbutamol is an effective way of lowering the serum potassium.
    D. an infusion of dextrose and insulin can reduce the serum potassium.
    E. dialysis can be effective treatment in severe cases.

23. **The following would be consistent with a diagnosis of Munchausen's syndrome by proxy (MSBP):**
    A. placing a thermometer in a cup of tea to elevate the temperature measurement.
    B. partially asphyxiating a child until apnoea occurs.
    C. persistent complaints of hyperactivity and poor sleeping.
    D. adding salt to an infant's milk to cause hypernatraemia.
    E. reporting seizures which have not occurred.

24. **The following are associated with Munchausen's syndrome by proxy:**
    A. a poor understanding of the true signs and symptoms of an illness.
    B. acute symptoms developing while medical staff are present.
    C. social isolation in the perpetrator.
    D. a history of an unexplained disorder in a previous sibling.
    E. a tendency for the perpetrator to avoid medical attention.

21. **ABCE**

The original injury causes a degree of primary brain injury, which is irreversible with current therapy. However, secondary damage may occur because of hypoxia, hypotension and cerebral oedema. Early treatment aims to minimise secondary injury. Further assessment of the severity of the injury involves a history of the injury, examination for external signs of injury and of neurological signs. The *Glasgow Coma Scale* is a measure of conscious level; an alert individual scores 15, and a low score indicates brain injury which could require neurosurgical intervention.

22. **CDE**

Hyperkalaemia is a dangerous condition but it is rare for children to experience arrhythmia at levels below 7.0 mmol/L. Intravenous calcium should be administered in the presence of arrhythmia. If the cardiac rhythm is stable, intravenous salbutamol can bring down the potassium level promptly. Intravenous dextrose and insulin and alkalinisation of the blood are beneficial measures. In severe cases, dialysis may be necessary.

23. **ABDE**

Occasionally parents – usually the mother – will falsify the history, manipulate investigations or contaminate samples or impose injury in order to fabricate an illness. MSBP should not be confused with parental anxiety or disagreement regarding diagnosis.

24. **CD**

Individuals suffering MSBP may 'research' the disorders they fabricate and can have quite detailed knowledge; MSBP is more common in individuals who have worked in health care. MSBP is more likely to occur in an isolated individual and can be interpreted as an extreme form of attention seeking. Suspicion of MSBP should be aroused if there are recurrent (usually dangerous) unexplained signs or symptoms which never occur when directly observed. Perpetrators seek medical attention since that is the goal of their activities and may seem strangely content with proposals for prolonged hospitalisation or intense investigation. A history of a similar situation with previous children may raise further suspicion.

**25. The following measures are likely to reduce the risk of sudden infant death syndrome (SIDS):**
- **A.** avoidance of exposure to cigarette smoke.
- **B.** ensuring that the infant is well wrapped at all times of year.
- **C.** use of an apnoea monitor.
- **D.** use of the prone position for sleeping.
- **E.** breast feeding.

**26. The following are associated with SIDS:**
- **A.** a higher risk in infants of higher birth weight.
- **B.** a higher risk in boys.
- **C.** a minor respiratory infection in the 24 hours before death.
- **D.** diagnosis of an inborn error of metabolism on postmortem investigation in the majority of cases.
- **E.** extensive abnormalities of the brain, heart and lungs found at post-mortem.

**27. The following are accurate observations which may be useful in the resuscitation of a sick child:**
- **A.** body weight increases by 20% during the 1st year after birth.
- **B.** the head of an infant accounts for a higher proportion of body surface area than in an older child.
- **C.** the larynx of a child is positioned high and anterior relative to the position in an adult.
- **D.** as in the adult, the larynx is the narrowest part of the airway.
- **E.** a small reduction in airway calibre may severely impede ventilation in a child.

**28. The following are useful in the recognition of an acutely ill child:**
- **A.** 'grunting' is a sign of respiratory distress in an infant.
- **B.** a respiratory rate of 45 breaths/min is abnormal at any age.
- **C.** hypotension is an early sign of circulatory failure.
- **D.** agitation or drowsiness in a child with respiratory illness is indicative of respiratory failure.
- **E.** clinical examination will detect mild hypoxaemia more effectively than a pulse oximeter.

**25. AE**

Case control and cohort studies have identified a number of associations with SIDS. These include sleeping in a prone position, maternal cigarette smoking, lack of breast feeding and over-wrapping of the baby. Campaigns to counter these risk factors have been associated with a fall in the incidence of SIDS in several countries. Apnoea monitors have not been conclusively proven to prevent SIDS cases.

**26. BC**

Sudden death is commoner in male infants and in those with a history of prematurity, low birth weight, multiple births and social disadvantage. In many cases, there is a history of minor respiratory infection in the preceding 24 hours. In a few cases, a specific diagnosis, such as an inborn error of metabolism or significant congenital abnormality, is discovered during post-mortem investigation, thus excluding a final diagnosis of SIDS.

**27. BCE**

A number of important anatomical and physiological differences between adults and children affect resuscitation techniques. Body weight increases rapidly during the first year from 3.5 kg at birth to approximately 10 kg by 1 year. The infant's head is relatively large compared to the body and differences in head and neck anatomy can make intubation more difficult. In a child the narrowest part of the airway is at the cricoid ring, below the larynx. Airflow is proportional to the 4th power of the radius, thus infants are especially vulnerable to any reduction in airway diameter.

**28. AD**

In paediatric practice, it is important to be aware of the normal ranges of respiratory rate, heart rate and blood pressure at different ages. Healthy infants may have respiratory rates of 40–60 breaths/min. Tachycardia and pallor are earlier signs of circulatory failure than hypotension. Cerebral abnormalities in a child with a respiratory disorder indicate hypoxaemia and/or hypercapnoea. Pulse oximeters are particularly useful in detecting mild hypoxaemia, which can be missed during physical examination.

29. **In the practice of paediatric intensive care the following principles apply:**
    A. an intensive care nurse should care for between three and six patients.
    B. open visiting by parents is likely to improve cooperation of the child.
    C. drug doses are usually calculated according to age.
    D. care is likely to be of a higher standard if delivered in a dedicated paediatric unit.
    E. unlike adults, sedation is unnecessary for most children receiving mechanical ventilation.

30. **When mechanically ventilating a 3-year-old child:**
    A. a cuffed endotracheal tube should be employed.
    B. a pulse oximeter is a reliable guide to the adequacy of oxygenation.
    C. an adequate oxygen saturation obviates the need for measurement of arterial $PCO_2$.
    D. regular suction of the endotracheal tube is likely to be necessary.
    E. humidification of the inspired gases is unnecessary.

**29.  BD**

One of the most important features of an intensive care unit is that there is a high nurse-to-patient ratio, typically one nurse for one or two patients. There is evidence that outcomes are improved if children are cared for in a dedicated paediatric unit, although financial or geographical limitations sometimes dictate that children are treated in adult ICUs. Drug doses are usually calculated according to body weight.

**30.  BD**

Inflatable cuffs are used to ensure a good seal around an endotracheal tube. Cuffed tubes are too bulky to be used in infants and young children. Although they have limitations, pulse oximeters are good indicators of adequate oxygenation but they give no information on pH or $PCO_2$ and measurement of arterial blood gases may be necessary in some cases. Continuing care of the airway is important, including suction to remove secretions and humidification of the gases to prevent drying of secretions and to protect the respiratory mucosa.

# MCQ Exam

1. **In severe congenital cytomegalovirus (CMV) infection:**
   A. there will always have been a primary maternal CMV infection during the pregnancy.
   B. there is symmetrical growth retardation of head circumference, body length and weight.
   C. there will be hepatosplenomegaly.
   D. a major cardiac malformation will be present.
   E. there will be a bleeding tendency in the first few days of life.

2. **Respiratory difficulty in the first 24 hours of life:**
   A. affects all babies born at less than 28 weeks' gestation.
   B. occurs more commonly in preterm boys than girls.
   C. is more likely after elective caesarean section than normal vaginal delivery.
   D. occurs if amniotic fluid enters the lower respiratory tract at delivery.
   E. is associated with a prolonged leak of amniotic fluid during pregnancy.

3. **Infecting organisms associated with neonatal septicaemia include:**
   A. *Streptococcus pneumoniae.*
   B. *Haemophilus influenzae.*
   C. *Mycoplasma pneumoniae.*
   D. group A beta-haemolytic Streptococci.
   E. *Escherichia coli.*

4. **Physiological jaundice on the 3rd day of life:**
   A. is due to an unconjugated hyperbilirubinaemia.
   B. occurs in less than 20% of full-term babies.
   C. is more common in breast-fed than bottle-fed infants.
   D. is most effectively treated by increasing the baby's fluid intake.
   E. is an indication to stop breast feeding.

1. **ACE**

Damaging congenital cytomegalovirus (CMV) infection only occurs if a mother develops her primary CMV infection during pregnancy. Reactivation of CMV infection rarely if ever leads to generalised fetal infection. In severe disease there is widespread tissue infection characterised by growth retardation, micro-cephaly, hepatosplenomegaly, thrombocytopenia and a degree of DIC are common. Major cardiac malformations are common in congenital rubella infection but not CMV.

2. **BCDE**

Not all babies born prematurely will suffer respiratory distress syndrome (RDS). RDS is commoner in boys than girls of the same gestation because male sex hormones have a maturation-retarding effect. Elective caesarean section is associated with delayed clearance of lung fluid and the resulting transient tachypnoea of the newborn (TTN) occurs more frequently than after normal delivery. Amniotic fluid (blood or meconium) breathed into the airways is an irritant and will cause respiratory difficulty. A prolonged leak of liquor for several months prior to delivery may be associated with pulmonary hypoplasia due to chest wall compression.

3. **E**

Common causes of neonatal septicaemia include group B beta-haemolytic Streptococci and *E. coli*. Less common causes include *S. aureus* and Listeria monocytogenes. Coagulase negative Staphylococci are important pathogens in the neonatal intensive-care setting. Mycoplasma and Ureaplasma infections may be associated with chronic lung disease in premature babies.

4. **AC**

Visible jaundice (bilirubin levels above 70 μmol/L) affects 60% of healthy term babies. Increased red cell breakdown and immaturity of the hepatic glucuronyl transferase results in an unconjugated hyperbilirubinaemia. Breast-fed babies do be-come more jaundiced than bottle-fed babies, but this is neither an indication for feeding additional water nor for discontinu-ing breast feeding. The condition is almost always benign and so long as the babies are healthy there is no need for further treatment, unless there is evidence of active haemolysis.

5. **Neonatal hypoglycaemia is associated with:**
   A. intrauterine growth retardation.
   B. prematurity.
   C. intrapartum asphyxia.
   D. breast feeding.
   E. high birthweight (> 4.5 kg).

6. **In simple obesity:**
   A. the height is greater than expected for age.
   B. the bone age will be retarded.
   C. striae do not occur.
   D. an underlying endocrine abnormality is commonly found.
   E. affected children are more likely to have affluent parents.

7. **Rectal blood loss is associated with:**
   A. accidental iron ingestion (overdose).
   B. a Meckel's diverticulum.
   C. ileocolic intussusception.
   D. coeliac disease.
   E. Campylobacter gastroenteritis.

8. **The following conditions are associated with intussusception:**
   A. cystic fibrosis.
   B. Henoch Schönlein purpura.
   C. intestinal polyposis.
   D. ulcerative colitis.
   E. pyloric stenosis.

**5. ABCE**

Liver glycogen and subcutaneous fat stores are laid down by the fetus over the last trimester of pregnancy, assuming there is adequate intrauterine nutrition. Therefore in premature babies (who may miss out on the last trimester), growth-retarded babies (who are starved) and asphyxiated babies (who are severely stressed) hypoglycaemia should be expected. Macrosomic babies may be stressed by a difficult labour and may be large as a result of fetal hyperinsulinism because of maternal gestational diabetes. Higher than normal blood glucose levels in utero trigger increased levels of fetal insulin, which is a growth-promoting hormone. Breast-fed babies should not develop significant hypoglycaemia.

**6. A**

Simple obesity is due to a combination of increased calorie intake and decreased calorie expenditure. Bone age is usually advanced and children are taller than expected for chronological age. The development of striae is associated with rapid weight gain and is not necessarily associated with excess endogenous or exogenous steroid. There is an inverse relationship between socio-economic status and the prevalence of obesity. Endocrine abnormality causing obesity is rare; however, obesity and short stature is an important combination suggesting endocrine disease.

**7. ABCE**

Iron poisoning may cause gastritis and bowel mucosal ulceration. A Meckel's diverticulum may be lined with gastric acid secreting mucosa, causing ulceration and haemorrhage. The intussusceptum (prolapsing portion of bowel) may become congested and ischaemic, resulting in the passage of bloody mucus – 'redcurrant jelly stool'. This is a late sign. Campylobacter, *E. coli*, Salmonella and Shigella enteritis may all cause rectal bleeding. Coeliac disease does not cause rectal bleeding.

**8. ABC**

Focal pathology is usually not present at the lead point of an intussusception. However, when present as in cystic fibrosis (adherent sticky faecal masses), in Henoch Schönlein purpura (haemorrhage into the bowel wall) or intestinal polyposis, such focal pathology may be an important trigger factor.

9. **Deficiency of the following vitamins is causally related to the medical conditions given below:**
   A. vitamin D and rickets.
   B. thiamine and dental caries.
   C. maternal folic acid deficiency and fetal neural tube defects.
   D. vitamin $B_{12}$ and microcytic anaemia.
   E. pyridoxine and intractable seizures in infancy.

10. **Jaundice and pale stools would be compatible with a diagnosis of:**
    A. breast-feeding jaundice.
    B. biliary atresia.
    C. choledochal cyst.
    D. cystic fibrosis.
    E. acute infectious hepatitis.

11. **Complications of gastro-oesphageal reflux include:**
    A. apnoea.
    B. recurrent pneumonia.
    C. haematemesis.
    D. failure to thrive.
    E. hypoglycaemia.

12. **Symptoms of heart failure in infancy include:**
    A. persistent vomiting.
    B. failure to thrive.
    C. persistent cough.
    D. slow feeding.
    E. lethargy.

**9.  ACE**

Dietary deficiency of vitamin D and calcium is the commonest and most easily treated form of rickets. Thiamine deficiency causes beriberi. Pellagra is caused by nicotinic acid (niacin) deficiency. Vitamin $B_{12}$ deficiency is usually associated with a macrocytic anaemia. Folic acid supplementation preconceptually has been shown virtually to eliminate the risk of spina bifida and anencephaly. Pyridoxine (Vitamin $B_6$) deficiency is associated with intractable neonatal seizures which respond promptly to the administration of intravenous pyridoxine.

**10.  BCDE**

Obstructive jaundice is characterised by pale stools, dark urine and green/yellow jaundice caused by a predominantly conjugated hyperbilirubinaemia. The jaundice associated with breast feeding is unconjugated as a result of immature conjugating enzymes and highly efficient enterohepatic circulation of bile. The other answers are all associated with intra- or post-hepatic cholestasis.

**11.  ABCD**

Gastric acid reflux into the oesophagus may cause reflex vagal-induced apnoea. Acid refluxing up to the larynx may cause vocal cord spasm and obstructive apnoea. Stomach contents aspirated repeatedly into the airway may cause recurrent chest infections. Oesophagitis may present as a haematemesis. Recurrent severe vomiting may result in failure to thrive, but the majority of babies with reflux gain weight satisfactorily. Unless the baby is profoundly malnourished, reflux will not cause hypoglycaemia.

**12.  ABCDE**

Breathlessness caused by heart failure results in poor feeding, poor calorie intake, excessive calorie consumption, lethargy and failure to thrive. Venous congestion of the bowel wall and liver may be responsible for recurrent vomiting and pulmonary congestion for a tendency to cough and a susceptibility to respiratory infections.

13. **Causes of cardiac failure in the 1st week of life include:**
    A. atrial septal defect.
    B. moderate pulmonary stenosis.
    C. complete heart block.
    D. Fallot's tetralogy.
    E. hypoplastic left heart.

14. **In congenital cyanotic heart disease:**
    A. cyanosis can be detected clinically only if the $PaO_2$ is less than 5 Kpa.
    B. all affected children are breathless at rest.
    C. breathing 100% oxygen will return the $PaO_2$ to normal.
    D. there is a significant left to right shunt.
    E. there will be a loud systolic murmur.

15. **The following findings would be more suggestive of a significant murmur than an innocent murmur:**
    A. a continuous murmur in the second right intercostal space which disappears on lying flat.
    B. a grade 2/6 systolic murmur.
    C. the presence of a thrill.
    D. splitting of the second heart sound.
    E. an increase in the loudness of a murmur after exercise.

16. **Causes of hypertension in a 2-year-old girl include:**
    A. neuroblastoma.
    B. minimal change nephrotic syndrome.
    C. coarctation of the aorta.
    D. reflux nephropathy.
    E. ventricular septal defect.

13. **CE**

Heart failure in the 1st week of life is rarely caused by left to right shunts due to the persistence of a high pulmonary vascular resistance under these circumstances. Severe obstructive lesions, e.g. coarctation, critical valve stenosis or atresia, or left ventricular hypoplasia, or major rhythm disturbances, e.g. tachy or severe brady arrhythmias, are the usual cause of early-onset heart failure.

14. **All false**

Clinically detectable cyanosis indicates that there is more than 5 g of deoxygenated Hb/100 ml blood in the skin capillaries. The $PaO_2$ at which this occurs will depend on the position of the oxygen dissociation curve. Children become breathless with hypoxia if there is a rapid fall in $PaO_2$, if tissue oxygenation is inadequate causing acidosis or if there is coexisting lung disease. Most children with congenital cyanotic heart disease are not breathless at rest. Left to right shunts are not associated with cyanosis. There may be no murmur in a child with cyanosis – e.g. in transposition of the great vessels the praecordium is commonly quiet on auscultation.

15. **C**

Murmurs associated with a thrill (grade IV), murmurs which radiate, and diastolic murmurs are all likely to be significant. A venous hum may be heard as a continuous murmur which disappears on lying down. The second heart sound is usually split, and the splitting increases with inspiration and reduces with expiration. A fixed split second sound is suggestive of an atrial septal defect. An innocent murmur may increase in intensity if the cardiac output is increased by fever or exercise.

16. **ACD**

Neuroblastomas may secrete catecholamines and cause hypertension. Minimal change nephrotic syndrome is not usually associated with hypertension. Coarctation of the aorta may cause hypertension in the upper limbs – a difference between upper- and lower-limb systolic pressure of more than 15 mmHg is significant. Renal scarring is a common cause of hypertension in children.

17. **A urinary tract infection:**
    A. can be diagnosed only with certainty when increased numbers of white cells are seen on microscopy of the urine.
    B. can be diagnosed if more than $10^5$ organisms are cultured in pure growth from a mid-stream urine sample.
    C. with mixed organisms obtained on culture is indicative of contamination of the sample.
    D. occurs as a result of haematogenous spread of bacteria to the renal tract.
    E. is usually diagnosed in children as a result of primary enuresis.

18. **Nocturnal enuresis in 5-year-olds:**
    A. is commoner in girls than boys.
    B. affects 20% of children aged 5.
    C. can be treated with evening fluid restriction.
    D. is effectively treated in at least 30% by bedtime administration of vasopressin analogues.
    E. is usually associated with daytime wetting.

19. **Typical findings in the nephrotic syndrome in children include:**
    A. haematuria.
    B. hypoalbuminuria.
    C. hypertension.
    D. raised levels of triglyceride and cholesterol.
    E. neutropenia.

20. **Hyperkalaemia:**
    A. is a feature of acute renal failure.
    B. causes inverted T-waves on ECG.
    C. is a feature of Addisonian crisis.
    D. causes multifocal ventricular ectopic beats.
    E. may be treated in the short term with intravenous salbutamol.

17.  **BC**

Urinary leukocytosis though common is not mandatory for the diagnosis of a urinary tract infection (UTI). In a mid-stream urine sample more than $10^5$ organisms per millilitre in pure growth are diagnostic of a UTI. In a suprapubic aspirate sample of urine a growth of $10^3$ organisms per millilitre is significant. A growth of mixed organisms on culture usually results from sample contamination, but if repeatedly obtained, then urinary obstruction should be suspected. Infection of the urinary tract is by ascending infection. Primary enuresis is rarely caused by long-standing undiagnosed UTI. Secondary enuresis is more likely to be associated with UTI.

18.  **CD**

In most aspects of development in childhood boys are less advanced than girls! At all ages enuresis is less common in girls than boys. By 5 years of age only 10% of children are still regularly wet at night. Approximately 15% become dry each year thereafter. Desmopressin may be effective in up to 50% of children in preventing nocturnal enuresis. Although evening fluid restriction and late night lifting with toileting can be effective, they have usually been tried by parents before they present for medical advice. Most children are dry by day by 3 years of age.

19.  **D**

Haematuria and hypertension are more typical of nephritis than minimal change nephrotic syndrome, which accounts for over 95% of childhood nephrosis. Neutropenia is not a feature. Hyperlipidaemia with oedema and hypoproteinaemia secondary to gross proteinuria are characteristic features of the nephrotic syndrome.

20.  **ACDE**

Hyperkalaemia is an important and potentially life-threatening complication of acute renal failure. Potassium levels above 6 mmol/L may be associated with tall, peaked T-waves on the ECG. Myocardial irritability is characterised by multifocal ventricular ectopic beats. Broadening of the QRS complex occurs before ventricular fibrillation. Hyponatraemia and hyperkalaemia are characteristic of Addison's disease. Treatments for hyperkalaemia include insulin and dextrose, intravenous calcium, bicarbonate, ion exchange resin, salbutamol and dialysis.

21. **Side-effects of long-term steroid therapy include:**
    A. cataracts.
    B. infertility.
    C. growth acceleration.
    D. ulceration of the large bowel.
    E. adrenal suppression.

22. **Hypoglycaemia is associated with the following conditions:**
    A. febrile convulsions.
    B. glycogen storage disorders.
    C. mucopolysaccharidoses.
    D. hypothyroidism.
    E. fatty acid oxidation defects.

23. **Breast development is seen in:**
    A. isolated premature thelarche.
    B. normal pubertal males.
    C. adrenal tumours.
    D. children on long-term antibiotic prophylaxis for urinary tract infection.
    E. Klinefelter syndrome.

24. **Early onset of puberty is associated with:**
    A. a familial tendency.
    B. Turner syndrome.
    C. hypothyroidism.
    D. cystic fibrosis.
    E. diabetes mellitus.

25. **A 4-year-old boy's height and weight are both increasing along the 3rd centile:**
    A. he is failing to thrive.
    B. his height velocity will be on the 3rd centile.
    C. 97% of boys of the same age will be taller than this child.
    D. height velocity will usually increase over the next 5 years.
    E. his weight will be increasing by approximately 3.5 kg per year.

21.  **AE**

Cataracts, growth suppression, adrenal suppression and increased susceptibility to peptic ulceration of the stomach or duodenum (but not large bowel ulceration) are some of the recognised problems of long-term oral steroid therapy in children. Side-effects are minimised by constantly ensuring that the smallest possible dose of steroid is used to suppress unacceptable symptoms. Treatment is given on alternate days if possible.

22.  **BE**

After febrile seizures, the blood sugar is commonly elevated as a part of the stress response. In mucopolysaccharide storage disorders and hypothyroidism glycogen and fat metabolism are not affected, and hypoglycaemia is not a feature. In glycogen storage disorders and fatty acid oxidation defects there are problems with the liberation of glucose from the body energy stores and therefore hypoglycaemia may result after a period of fasting or under the metabolic stress of an infection.

23.  **ABCE**

Gynaecomastia is not uncommon in normal males and is common in up to 50% of males with Klinefelter syndrome (XXY) at puberty. In young girls under the age of 2 years isolated thelarche (without any other signs of precocious puberty) requires no further treatment and generally resolves. Rarely adrenal or ovarian tumours may produce oestrogen causing breast enlargement. Antibiotics have no effect on breast tissue in children.

24.  **AC**

A family history is important when considering the appropriate-ness of the timing of the onset of puberty. In Turner syndrome puberty will not occur without pharmacological assistance. In hypothyroidism puberty may be delayed or may be advanced if FSH and LH production is switched on with the elevation of TSH.

25.  **C**

A child whose height and weight are increasing along the 3rd centile is growing at a normal velocity and therefore is not failing to thrive. Height velocity will be slightly below the 50th centile. Height velocity decreases from birth to the onset of puberty. Normal weight gain after infancy and before the onset of puberty is 2–2.5 kg per year.

26. **A bone age that is 2 years behind chronological age:**
    A. is diagnostic of hypothyroidism.
    B. is a feature of constitutional growth delay.
    C. indicates that the final height will be greater than predicted from the parents' height.
    D. indicates that the onset of puberty may be delayed.
    E. gives an indication of the amount of potential growth remaining.

27. **Signs of early puberty include:**
    A. enlargement of the testes to greater than 4 ml volume.
    B. the onset of menstruation.
    C. peaking of pubertal growth velocity spurt.
    D. development of the breast bud.
    E. breaking of the voice in males.

28. **By 9 months, most infants will be able to:**
    A. stand holding on to the furniture.
    B. build a tower of 2 bricks.
    C. point to objects to indicate their needs.
    D. respond to their own name.
    E. feed with a spoon.

29. **Warning signs of abnormal development in a 6-month-old child include:**
    A. presence of grasp reflex.
    B. inability to sit unsupported.
    C. absence of polysyllabic babble ('mamama', 'dadada').
    D. development of right-hand preference.
    E. inability to swallow lumpy food without gagging and choking.

26. **BDE**

    A delayed or advanced bone age is not diagnostic of any particular condition, although the bone age may be delayed in hypothyroidism. This assessment gives only an indication of the remaining growth potential. The bone age will be delayed in constitutional growth delay, and if delayed by 2 years in early adolescence, it is likely to be associated with a delay in the onset of puberty. Predictions of final height cannot be made from the information given.

27. **AD**

    Enlargement of the testes to 3–4 ml size and enlargement of the breasts to form a breast bud are the earliest signs of the onset of puberty in boys and girls respectively. Menstruation, peak growth velocity and change in the character of the voice (in males) all occur late in puberty.

28. **AD**

    By 9 months most infants will not be able to pull up to stand, but they will stand holding on. They will reach out for small objects with an index finger approach but will not yet have a neat pincer grip. They will not point at objects until 12–13 months. They will not yet have a hand preference. They will not yet be able to feed themselves with a spoon, but will finger feed. They will not be able to build towers of bricks, but may respond to their own name. They will turn their head readily to sounds.

29. **AD**

    The grasp reflex should disappear before an infant is able to develop hand skills – by 6 months most infants reach out for objects and readily transfer. By 6 months, many infants will sit only with support. Single-syllable vocalising would be normal at 6 months, and polysyllabic babble should not be expected until around 9 months. Handedness does not develop until 18 months. Many children of 18 months and above are still having problems with lumpy food.

30. **The routine vaccination programme for children in the UK includes:**
    A. diphtheria, tetanus and pertussis (DTP) vaccination at 2, 3 and 4 months after the expected date of delivery.
    B. a booster dose of DTP before school entry.
    C. further doses of both polio and tetanus vaccines before leaving school.
    D. immunisation against chickenpox before school entry.
    E. rubella immunisation at 13 months and repeat dose for adolescent girls.

31. **The following vaccines contain live virus:**
    A. pertussis.
    B. oral polio.
    C. BCG.
    D. mumps.
    E. Hib.

32. **Complications of measles include:**
    A. thrombocytopenia.
    B. croup.
    C. gastroenteritis.
    D. encephalitis.
    E. late-onset developmental regression and fits.

33. **Patients at high risk after exposure to Varicella zoster (VZ) infection include:**
    A. asthmatics on inhaled steroids.
    B. babies born to VZ-immune mothers.
    C. children with hypogammaglobulinaemia.
    D. children with temporal lobe epilepsy.
    E. children receiving treatment for relapsing nephrotic syndrome.

**30.  C**

DTP immunisation is timed from birth and not from the expected date of delivery (EDD). Many premature babies will therefore receive their first doses of immunisation even before their EDD. Booster doses of pertussis vaccine are not required. There is no chickenpox immunisation programme in the UK. Rubella immunisation is routinely given only to adolescent girls if there is no documented evidence of them having received MMR vaccine in infancy. Rubella vaccine is given at 12–15 months and again preschool.

**31.  BCD**

Pertussis vaccine is a suspension of killed *B. pertussis* organisms. Newer acellular vaccines have been produced and appear to have a reduced risk of side-effects. Oral polio vaccine contains live attenuated strains of polio virus types 1, 2 and 3. BCG vaccine contains live attenuated vaccine derived from *Mycobacterium bovis*. Mumps vaccine contains live attenuated vaccine. Hib vaccine contains capsular polysaccharide antigen only.

**32.  ABCDE – all of these**

Upper airway obstruction due to tracheobronchitis in measles is one of the commoner causes of deaths from measles in the UK. Gastroenteritis is common. Post-infectious encephalitis may result from direct brain infection or as a result of an (auto)immune process resulting in demyelination. Sub-acute sclerosing panencephalitis is a late-onset degenerative condition following previous measles infection. Significant thrombocytopenia occasionally occurs.

**33.  CE**

Inhaled steroids are not immunosuppressant. Children at high risk include neonates (with non-immune mothers), children receiving chemotherapy and children with antibody or cell-mediated immunity defects. Oral steroids in high dose will cause immunosuppression (>2 mg/kg for more than 1 week in the preceding 3 months) and patients may be at risk of disseminated VZ disease. Zoster-immune globulin should be given to at-risk patients as soon as possible after exposure.

**34. An increased risk of pneumococcal infection is associated with:**
   A. relapsed nephrotic syndrome.
   B. splenectomy.
   C. sickle cell disease.
   D. thalassaemia.
   E. cystic fibrosis.

**35. The following skin conditions can be expected to resolve without treatment:**
   A. capillary haemangioma (port wine stain).
   B. pigmented hairy naevus.
   C. café au lait patch.
   D. mongolian blue spot.
   E. strawberry naevus.

**36. Vesicular eruptions are a feature of the following conditions:**
   A. scabies.
   B. measles.
   C. eczema herpeticum.
   D. candidal napkin dermatitis.
   E. insect bites.

**37. Condylomata acuminata:**
   A. lesions may be seen on the face, flexures and trunk.
   B. are caused by the human pox virus.
   C. are easily transmissible by normal social contact.
   D. occur only following child sexual abuse.
   E. are usually asymptomatic.

34. **ABC**

Nephrotic syndrome in relapse is associated with a high risk of pneumococcal infection. Children after splenectomy and those at risk of auto-splenectomy, as occurs in sickle cell disease, are also at high risk. There is no increased risk of pneumococcal infection in thalassaemia, and children with cystic fibrosis are rarely affected by pneumococci.

35. **DE**

Capillary haemangiomas do not resolve, but may be effectively treated with laser therapy. Pigmented naevi do not resolve and are best treated by excision and grafting. Café au lait patches do not resolve and increase in number during childhood in neurofibromatosis type 1. Mongolian blue spots, an accumulation of melanocytes deep within the dermis, are usually seen over the lumbar-sacral region. They fade before the age of 7 years. Strawberry naevi increase in size over the first few months of life, epithelialise during the second 6 months of life and resolve leaving only a few superficial capillary vessels by the end of the 2nd year.

36. **ACE**

Scabies is an itchy papular or vesicular eruption. Measles has an erythematous maculo-papular rash. Eczema is exacerbated usually by bacterial infection but occasionally by Herpes simplex – suggested by the presence of vesicles. T-cell function is abnormal in eczema. Herpes infection may therefore become generalised and systemic treatment with acyclovir should be started. Insect bites are usually papular but may become vesicular or bullous as a result of the allergic response to the bite. Candida nappy rash is erythematous with satellite lesions, and involves skin flexures, but is not usually vesicular.

37. **E**

Condylomata acuminata, or venereal warts, are caused by the human papilloma virus. The virus is only transmitted by close contact, commonly sexual contact in adolescents. Close family contact is thought to be a means of transmission in young children. Neonatal transmission has been documented. Most lesions are asymptomatic unless traumatised or secondarily infected. The warts are usually present around the posterior vaginal introitus and/or perianal regions.

38. **The following *neonatal* skin conditions usually require no investigation or treatment:**
    A. erythema toxicum.
    B. neonatal acne.
    C. naevus flammeus – salmon patch.
    D. milia.
    E. bullous skin eruptions.

39. **Recognised risk factors for congenital dislocation of the hip include:**
    A. prolonged labour.
    B. oligohydramnios.
    C. male sex.
    D. hypertonic cerebral palsy.
    E. premature delivery.

40. **The following features would be more in keeping with a diagnosis of a septic arthritis rather than of an 'irritable hip' (transient synovitis):**
    A. ESR 100 mm/hour.
    B. reluctance to walk.
    C. joint effusion seen on ultrasound scan.
    D. turbid fluid on joint aspiration.
    E. elevated peripheral blood neutrophil count.

41. **Structural scoliosis in childhood:**
    A. most commonly affects females.
    B. is usually associated with an underlying vertebral or muscular abnormality.
    C. is associated with rotation of the vertebrae.
    D. will disappear on bending forward to touch the toes.
    E. usually causes more than one curve of the spine.

38. **ABCD**

Erythema toxicum/neonatorum is a common, benign, erythematous, papular skin eruption seen during the first 10 days of life. Neonatal acne is common in the first few weeks of life, due to maternal androgens, and requires no treatment. The naevus flammeus, or stork mark, results from dilated superficial capillaries over the forehead, bridge of the nose, eyelids and the nape of the neck; it usually fades by one year. Milia are spontaneously resolving, small, whitish-yellow papules seen on the face of neonates; they are tiny epithelial cysts arising from hair follicles. Neonatal bullous skin eruptions should be vigorously investigated and treatment for suspected Staphylococcal infection started immediately. If cultures are negative and new bullae continue to form, a skin biopsy may be necessary – suspect one of the congenital blistering skin disorders.

39. **B**

Female sex, breech position during pregnancy, family history, oligohydramnios and neuromuscular disorders are all considered to be risk factors for congenital hip dislocation. Prolonged or premature labour have no such association. While children with cerebral palsy with hypertonus of the hip adductors are at risk of hip dislocation, this is an acquired rather than congenital problem.

40. **AE**

A raised peripheral blood white cell count and high ESR would be consistent with a diagnosis of septic arthritis. Reluctance to walk and a joint effusion seen on ultrasound scan could be present in either condition. Turbid synovial fluid would also not be discriminatory as raised numbers of WBC in the synovial fluid occur in both conditions. Culture of synovial would be positive in septic arthritis.

41. **ACE**

Scoliosis affects girls more commonly than boys and is most commonly idiopathic. A scoliosis will usually show a double S-shaped curve of the spine, in association with rotation of vertebrae around their vertical axis, producing a rib hump posteriorly. A non-structural or compensatory scoliosis will disappear on forward flexion.

42. **Signs and symptoms of rickets include:**
    A. a proximal myopathy.
    B. microcephaly.
    C. defective tooth enamel.
    D. knock knees (genu valgus).
    E. deformity of the chest.

43. **Features of Henoch Schönlein purpura include:**
    A. thrombocytopenia.
    B. colicky abdominal pain.
    C. an urticarial rash which may precede the development of purpura.
    D. arthritis involving the small joints of the hands and feet.
    E. an increased risk of intussusception.

44. **Thrombocytopenia is a recognised complication of the following conditions:**
    A. meningococcal septicaemia.
    B. hypersplenism.
    C. acute myeloid leukaemia.
    D. haemophilia A.
    E. cavernous haemangioma.

45. **A prolonged bleeding time is seen in:**
    A. factor-8 deficiency disease.
    B. disseminated intravascular coagulation.
    C. von Willebrand's disease.
    D. aspirin therapy.
    E. heparin therapy.

42.  **ACDE**
In rickets there may be a proximal myopathy. There may be the appearance of macrocephaly with frontal bossing of the skull. Bone abnormality may result in bow legs (genu varus) or knock knees (genu valgus), expansion of the ends of the ribs (rickety rosary) and deformity of the chest with pectus excavatum and/ or Harrison's sulcus. Abnormal calcium metabolism during teeth formation may lead to abnormal enamel formation.

43.  **BCE**
Henoch Schönlein purpura is a vasculitic condition which commonly involves the skin, gut, joints and less frequently the kidneys. An urticarial skin rash over the legs commonly precedes the purpuric rash. The platelet count is normal. There is often quite marked soft tissue swelling over the dorsum of the feet and around the ankles. Large joints only are involved, often only transiently. Vasculitis affecting the gut may cause colicky abdominal pain and some rectal bleeding. There may be evidence of bowel wall ischaemia. Intussusception may occur and can be readily diagnosed by ultrasound examination.

44.  **ABCE**
Platelets may be consumed by intravascular coagulation in meningococcaemia and in the abnormal circulation of a large cavernous haemangioma. In conditions associated with hypersplenism, there will be sequestration of platelets and possibly also white cells and red cells in the spleen. In any condition associated with infiltration of the bone marrow, platelet numbers will fall if megakaryocytes are displaced. Platelet numbers fall early in leukaemia, often before blast cells appear in the peripheral blood. Platelet numbers are normal in haemophilia.

45.  **BCD**
A prolonged bleeding time is seen where there is abnormality of platelet function or numbers, or where there is abnormal vessel wall function. In haemophilia platelet numbers and function are normal in contrast with von Willebrand's disease where there is reduced platelet aggregation, as well as abnormal factor-8 levels. Aspirin is used therapeutically to reduce platelet adhesiveness. Heparin exerts its anticoagulant effect by potentiating the activity of antithrombin III – platelet function is unaffected.

46. **Complications of sickle cell disease include:**
    A. mental retardation.
    B. avascular necrosis of the femoral head.
    C. osteomyelitis.
    D. haemolysis with administration of oxidant drugs.
    E. acute hemiparesis.

47. **Haemolysis is associated with:**
    A. abnormalities of red cell shape.
    B. reduction of red cell iron content.
    C. increased sensitivity of the red cells to osmotic lysis.
    D. antioxidant deficiency.
    E. chronic hypoxia.

48. **Neuroblastoma in childhood:**
    A. is the commonest solid tumour occurring outside the central nervous system.
    B. has a uniformly poor prognosis.
    C. may regress spontaneously.
    D. commonly metastasises to bone.
    E. may present in infancy with massive hepatomegaly with good prognosis.

49. **Side-effects of current treatment for good-prognosis leukaemia include:**
    A. transient alopecia.
    B. thrombocytopenia.
    C. male infertility.
    D. growth failure.
    E. learning disability.

**46.   BCE**

Sickle cell disease vaso-occlusive complications affecting bones include dactylitis, bone pain and avascular necrosis of the femoral head. Osteomyelitis especially affects the under-5s. Salmonella is the infecting organism in over 50% of cases. CNS involvement is seen in 5% of patients and includes acute hemiparesis. There is no direct effect of the disease on IQ. Drugs do not induce acute haemolysis.

**47.   ACD**

Any abnormality of red cell shape results in increased red cell osmotic fragility. Cell membranes are protected against oxidant damage by a variety of antioxidants, including vitamin E, deficiency of which may result in a haemolytic anaemia. Chronic hypoxia increases red cell numbers. Iron deficiency does not cause haemolysis.

**48.   ACDE**

Brain tumours are the commonest group of solid tumours in childhood, but neuroblastoma is the commonest single type of solid tumour. Prognosis varies with tumour stage and age at diagnosis. Stage I or II disease has up to 90% cure rate with surgery alone. Patients with stage IV disease have at best a 20% chance of long-term survival. Some tumours may regress spontaneously. There is a special type of neuroblastoma – i.e. stage IV-S – in which there may be massive liver enlargement but no bony metastases in which there is a good chance of spontaneous regression of the tumour without therapy.

**49.   AB**

Baldness is an unavoidable but reversible side-effect of most treatments for cancer in childhood. Thrombocytopenia and neutropenia are common after courses of treatment, and may also require treatment. Male infertility does not usually occur in this tumour group. Growth failure and learning difficulty was found after cranial irradiation but this is no longer a part of the routine treatment of good-prognosis ALL.

50. **Clinical features of a cerebellar astrocytoma in childhood include:**
    A. ataxia.
    B. focal seizures.
    C. visual field defect.
    D. recurrent vomiting.
    E. growth failure.

51. **Marked lymphocytosis in the peripheral blood may be found:**
    A. following a febrile convulsion.
    B. in established whooping cough.
    C. in Hodgkin's lymphoma.
    D. in pulmonary tuberculosis.
    E. in severe chronic eczema.

52. **A 3-year-old child has swallowed an unknown quantity of turps substitute (white spirit). Treatment should include:**
    A. induction of vomiting with ipecac.
    B. gastric lavage with a cuffed endotracheal tube.
    C. oral administration of activated charcoal.
    D. careful monitoring of coagulation and liver function over the next 4 days.
    E. reassurance of the parents, and if the child is asymptomatic, discharge home without admission.

53. **Sudden infant death syndrome:**
    A. affects 1 in 200 infants under 1 year of age.
    B. may be prevented by prone lying.
    C. is commoner in the winter months.
    D. has double the risk of recurrence in siblings born after the index case.
    E. is often caused by inhalation of vomit.

50. **AD**

Do not be put off by mention of esoteric cerebellar astrocytomas! Most brain tumours in children occur below the tentorium – in the posterior fossa. Focal seizures are therefore uncommon. Raised intracranial pressure is suggested by recurrent vomiting and ataxia. A visual field defect and growth failure may be associated with a craniopharyngioma – one of the commoner types of supratentorial tumours in childhood.

51. **All false**

Following severe stress, such as a febrile convulsion, a *neutrophil* leukocytosis is a common finding. A lymphocytosis is characteristic of the *prodromal* stage of pertussis infection and has usually resolved by the time the paroxysmal cough is established. The blood count is then unhelpful in diagnosis. Peripheral blood examination will be unhelpful in the diagnosis of Hodgkin's disease and pulmonary tuberculosis. Children with eczema are likely to have an eosinophilia.

52. **All false**

After ingestion of turps substitute or white spirit, gastric lavage and induction of vomiting are contraindicated in order to minimise the risk of aspiration of hydrocarbon into the lungs (unless the hydrocarbons are themselves toxic – e.g. benzene, toluene, carbon tetrachloride or pesticides). Activated charcoal is of no benefit. There is minimal risk of liver dysfunction. Children should be admitted for observation as respiratory difficulty may develop up to 12 hours after ingestion.

53. **C**

Sudden infant death syndrome used to affect 2 infants per 1000 births, with most deaths occurring between 2 and 6 months. Since mothers have been advised to put babies to sleep in the supine position, there has been a dramatic fall in the incidence. The mortality rate is increased in the winter months, and at postmortem a high proportion of babies are found to have had a mild respiratory infection. There is no strong evidence of a significantly increased risk to siblings. Cot death, by definition, has no adequate explanation and therefore inhalation of vomit is not a cause.

**54. Following a head injury:**

    **A.** a patient may safely be allowed home if there are no external signs of injury, is fully conscious and there has been no loss of consciousness at any time after the accident.

    **B.** a lumbar puncture should be performed to determine whether there is bloodstaining of the CSF.

    **C.** an intact corneal reflex indicates integrity of the trigeminal nerve.

    **D.** CSF otorrhoea always indicates the presence of a skull fracture.

    **E.** a CT scan should be performed in all patients who have suffered loss of consciousness.

**55. In carbon monoxide poisoning:**

    **A.** carbon monoxide binds irreversibly to haemoglobin.

    **B.** carbon monoxide inhibits tissue cytochrome oxidase.

    **C.** headache is a common symptom.

    **D.** cherry red discolouration of the lips is commonly seen.

    **E.** there will be a metabolic acidosis if there is a high level of carbon monoxide in the blood.

**56. The following congenital abnormalities and aetiological factors are causally linked:**

    **A.** microcephaly and maternal alcohol ingestion.

    **B.** cleft lip and maternal phenobarbitone anticonvulsant therapy.

    **C.** anencephaly and maternal vitamin $B_{12}$ deficiency.

    **D.** pulmonary stenosis and congenital rubella infection.

    **E.** Turner syndrome and increasing paternal age.

**57. In X-linked recessive genetic disease:**

    **A.** if mother is a carrier, 50% of all offspring will be affected.

    **B.** if mother is a carrier, all girls will be carriers.

    **C.** if father is affected, all girls will be carriers.

    **D.** if father is affected, all boys will be normal.

    **E.** females are as commonly affected as males.

**54.  CD**

A patient should be allowed home only after low-impact injury and if the patient's condition can be regularly monitored. A lumbar puncture (LP) should never be undertaken when there is a possibility of raised intracranial pressure. LP has no place in the diagnosis of head injury. It is not practicable to CT-scan all patients who have suffered a brief loss of consciousness. If there has been a major impact, if there is altered conscious level or abnormal signs on neurological examination, then CT scan should be performed urgently.

**55.  BCE**

Carbon monoxide (CO) inhibits the cytochrome oxidase system and binds to haemoglobin with a higher affinity than oxygen. The half-life of HbCO in 100% oxygen is around 1 hour. Headache, nausea, vomiting and ataxia precede mental confusion, coma and convulsions. The symptoms of CO poisoning arise as a result of tissue hypoxia, which will commonly be accompanied by a metabolic acidosis in the event of a severe poisoning episode. Cherry pink lips are rarely seen.

**56.  ABD**

Alcohol exposure in utero has a dose-related effect on the fetus. Growth retardation is common, together with disproportionate retardation of brain growth. Cleft lip is more common in mothers taking anticonvulsants in pregnancy. Neural tube defects are associated with a folic acid deficient diet. Rubella infection is associated with pulmonary stenosis, ventricular septal defect and persistent ductus arteriosus. Turner syndrome is not associated with increased maternal or paternal age.

**57.  CD**

A carrier mother will pass on her affected X chromosome to 50% of her offspring. 50% of the boys will therefore be affected, but unless the father also carries an abnormal X, none of the girls will be affected. If father is affected, he will pass on his (only) affected X chromosome to all of his daughters, who will therefore all be carriers, while he will pass on his Y chromosome to his sons, who will neither be carriers nor affected.

**58. The following conditions have an autosomal dominant mode of inheritance:**
 A. atopic eczema.
 B. pyloric stenosis.
 C. congenital dislocation of the hip.
 D. Turner syndrome.
 E. spherocytosis.

**59. In Down syndrome:**
 A. the majority of affected babies are born to mothers over the age of 40 years.
 B. babies all have single palmar creases.
 C. affected children are at increased risk of hypothyroidism.
 D. occurrence is sporadic with no increased risk of recurrence.
 E. karyotype is usually expressed as 46, XX or XY, +21.

**60. In physically injured infants:**
 A. the age of fractures can be accurately assessed by their X-ray appearances.
 B. retinal haemorrhages usually occur as a result of an impact head injury.
 C. posterior rib fractures are often found after a severe shaking injury.
 D. a depressed skull fracture in a 6-month-old child could reasonably be explained by a fall from a height of 3 ft on to a carpeted floor.
 E. most children with repeated fractures occurring over time have some form of brittle bone disease.

**58. E**

Atopic eczema has a multifactorial mode of inheritance in most cases. There are a few families in whom there does appear to be a dominant gene on chromosome 11. Pyloric stenosis and congenital dislocation of the hip have a familial tendency but not clear-cut Mendelian types of inheritance. Girls with Turner syndrome are sterile. Spherocytosis is an autosomal dominant characteristic.

**59. C**

Most babies, and therefore most Down syndrome babies, are delivered by younger mothers. Not all babies with Down syndrome have single palmar creases. There is an increased risk of autoimmune disease in Down syndrome. Hypothyroidism is difficult to diagnose clinically. All Down syndrome children should have their thyroid function checked annually. There is a significant risk of recurrence if there has already been one non-disjunction episode, or if either parent has a balanced translocation. Karyotype is usually expressed as 47, XX or XY, +21.

**60. C**

The ageing of fractures is performed by consideration of radiological evidence of healing. It is difficult to assess how recent or how old. Retinal haemorrhages usually occur as a result of a sudden increase in central venous pressure, usually as a result of the chest being squeezed. Posterior rib fractures are commonly found after a gripping/shaking injury of the chest. Children rarely sustain skull fractures in falls from household furniture. Only single, simple, linear parietal fractures are likely to be accidental. Osteogenesis imperfecta is rarely a cause of recurrent fractures, but it must be considered.

# Index